THE DIABETIC GOURMET

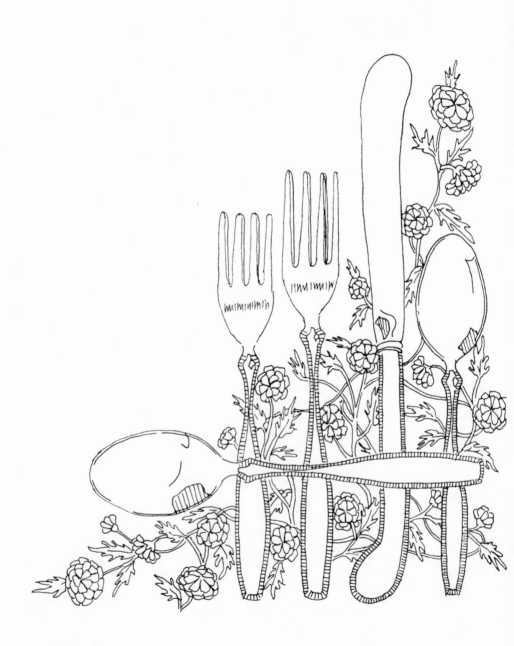

The Diabetic Gourmet

ANGELA BOWEN, M.D.

REVISED EDITION

with illustrations by Mary Pinckney Ferguson

HARPER & ROW, PUBLISHERS

NEW YORK

Cambridge
Hagerstown
Philadelphia
San Francisco

1817

London
Mexico City
São Paulo
Sydney

Designer: Sidney Feinberg

Library of Congress Cataloging in Publication Data

Bowen, Angela J   M   1932–
  The diabetic gourmet.
  Bibliography: p.
  Includes index.
  1. Diabetes—Diet therapy—Recipes. I. Title

RC662.B68 1980   641.5′63   79–1655
ISBN 0–06–010437–6

80 81 82 83 10 9 8 7 6 5 4 3 2

Contents

Preface

As this revision was begun, I sat down and reviewed the previous edition (one of the very few times I had picked it up since I wrote the book—you get really sick of reading your own book by the time the last galley is proofread!) to decide what needed to be changed. The inevitable answer was "almost all of it." Since the first edition was published in 1970, many changes have occurred in our understanding of the nutritional requirements of diabetics, in foods, in attitudes toward food, life styles, families, food preparation—and in me.

The opening line of my first Preface hit me soundly in the face with that reality. It read: "Housewives and mothers bear significant responsibility for maintaining the health of their families." How quaint that sounds in 1980, when it is common for fathers to plan and prepare meals, do the shopping, and have custody of the children.

Many of my colleagues warned me that I would be considered part of the lunatic fringe if I publicly advocated in the first edition the use of whole-grain cereals and breads, brewer's yeast, and wheat germ. Even to purchase such foods it was necessary to brave a trip to a "health food store" in 1970. Today you can buy them in your corner grocery because the demand permits that. Microwave ovens and food processors had not begun to work their magic in kitchens across the country, and those words did not appear in the first edition.

Some things have not changed. Doctors are still arguing about what is the "best" kind of diabetic diet, whether cholesterol intake really matters, whether sugar isn't really more hazardous to your health than either cyclamate or saccharin, and so on. We do not offer answers to any of those debates, and they will probably still be raging for the next edition!

But herein lies my approach to coping in 1980.

Acknowledgments

I am grateful to the many readers who took the time to write about what they found interesting, unsatisfactory, recipes that didn't work for them, errors, and bad prose. These have been invaluable in preparation of the revision.

Cathy Paullin, our dietitian, worried along with me about calories, calculations, and nutritional content and handled the drudgery of calculations singlehandedly.

Mary Pinckney Ferguson has again furnished the illustrations, moral support, and her unique sense of humor.

My husband proofread, criticized, helped, and encouraged until it was all done.

My family and friends have been patient in their willingness to sample innumerable variations of things that didn't quite work. Their participation in alterations that "might" taste better or be fluffier or hold longer approaches epic proportions.

Carol Van Auken has shopped, cleaned up after, tasted, and typed for months.

A cookbook is a lot of work. I hope you enjoy it.

THE DIABETIC GOURMET

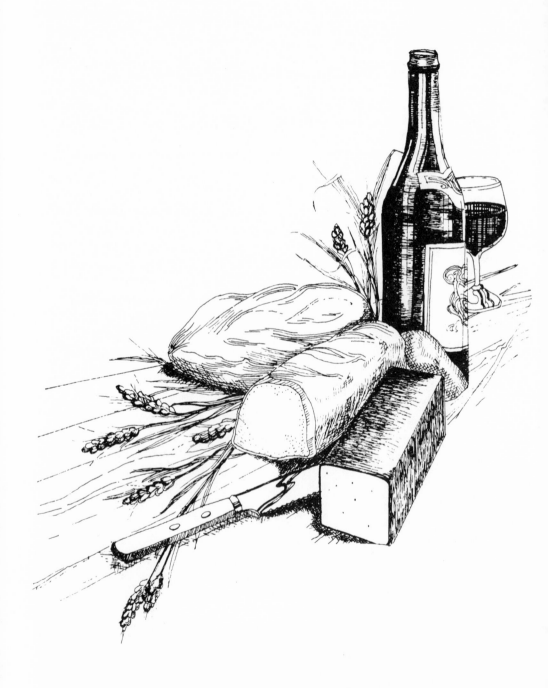

CHAPTER 1

Understanding Your Diet

Many variations of the diabetic diet have evolved over the years. Diabetic patients come in delightful variety: they are young, old, thin, fat, plump, anxious, calm, interested, and unconcerned. Obviously, the diet that is good for the plump fifty-five-year-old is not the same as is required for the growing youngster of eight. A severely diabetic juvenile requiring insulin may need to be on the strictest of diets, while the mildly diabetic normal-weight oldster can take a lot of liberties with his diet. In other words, a diet prescription is a very individual thing, and your physician will have taken many factors into account before prescribing. It is important, then, to stay with your own program. Don't recommend your diet to anyone else and don't be tempted by someone else's diet even though it may seem simpler.

Whatever your diet plan, the most important thing is that you understand it as completely as possible. Know the categories of foods that should be taken daily and the ones you should never have. If you can't understand it the way your doctor explains it, ask to be referred to a good consulting dietitian or nutritionist. Most hospitals have such people on their staff. Don't give up until a full understanding is acquired. A brief description of the commoner forms of diabetic diets follows.

SUGAR-FREE DIET

This is the simplest of the diabetic diets in general use and is usually limited to persons with very mild diabetes, those with normal weight, and those nondiabetics thought to have a high risk of developing the disease. This diet is simply one that avoids all sugar. Sugar is a kind of carbohydrate that is quickly absorbed into the bloodstream. Sugar includes not only the ordinary table variety but also honey, corn syrup, all foods with sugar added, some fruit juices, and a few of the fruits that are especially high in natural sugars. Carbohydrates other than sugar are not usually limited in a sugar-free diet. Bread is an example of a carbohydrate food that is not a sugar and that can be taken by a person on a sugar-free diet. It is not customary to have patients on these diets weigh or measure foods. They are especially well suited to the elderly.

ALTERED-FAT DIETS

There has been and continues to be such a wide difference of opinion among medical people concerning dietary fat that a prudent person hesitates to write about the subject. It must be difficult for the patient to understand how such wide differences continue to prevail, but there are, of course, reasons.

Our knowledge of the clinical disorders of fat metabolism is not yet complete. For years, clinicians have worried about cholesterol levels. It now appears that the fraction of fat called high-density lipoproteins (HDL) may be of more clinical importance than total cholesterol levels. And so it goes that we must continue to learn and change our minds when new evidence seems well enough established to warrant such a change.

We are still far from having a complete understanding of the most advantageous changes to make in fat intake. Each patient should make such changes as will keep the blood sugar, triglycerides, and cholesterol within a normal range. The principles outlined here will touch on the practical problems and potential pitfalls that a patient may encounter when a new diet prescription is put into effect. Unsaturated fat has been included in many recipes for those people who need to make this alteration. On the other hand, you will find butter and cream in many recipes, for we do not share the idea that *everyone* must forgo saturated fat.

One of the lessons learned over the past ten years in medical practice, particularly in nutrition, is that there is many a slip between what you have told a patient to do and what that patient does to follow those instructions. I shudder to think how many people gave up milk and cream in their coffee and substituted the nondairy creamers, which contain more saturated fat than good fresh cream. They advertise "no animal fat," and indeed it is so, but they use coconut oil instead, which is also saturated. It is true that they contain less cholesterol, but that adjustment could have been made using milk instead of cream. It is likewise appalling to find that many good, conscientious mothers are feeding their children a bowl of sweet cold cereal in the morning instead of the meat and eggs that were more common years ago. This, too, is often done in the spirit of trying to cut down cholesterol intake, but the net result has been to cut down protein intake and increase sugar intake.

I don't disagree with the theory of decreased fat intake, but I do disagree with the way it is put into practice. I see milk, and consequently calcium, omitted entirely from many diets, even children's diets, because skim milk is not enjoyed. I see eggs omitted entirely because of the cholesterol content, yet eggs provide a good source of protein and iron. The people who are evangelical about low-cholesterol diets may not be aware that their advice is interpreted in this manner, but in many cases it is.

Keep a careful record of a week's food intake for the diabetic patient in your family, and have your doctor or dietitian review it to be sure that nutritional needs are being met.

Blood cholesterol comes from two general sources: the cholesterol present in the foods we eat and that manufactured in our own body from other fats. Of these two sources the latter is much more important. Should we then omit all foods that contain much cholesterol? Not necessarily. Many disorders of fat metabolism are not measurably affected by eliminating all cholesterol from the diet. Others are affected. This must be determined on an individual basis. Unfortunately, strong statements, both pro and con, abound in medical and lay literature. The practicing physician is perhaps the best qualified to moderate these extremes as they are applied daily, and it is well to note that sometimes they work and sometimes they do not. Unfortunately, there are no definite answers at this time.

Many physicians feel that the fat allotment in the diets of all diabetics should consist only of highly unsaturated fat. Although this feeling is not universal, the fat allotment in all diets should include some unsaturated fat, preferably at least as much unsaturated as saturated fat. Stricter diets will require that at least 80 percent of fat calories be unsaturated. This is not the typical American diet, and if you are required to adhere to such a program, many changes will be in store! Such a diet will require special help from a dietitian or a nutritionist.

EXCHANGE DIETS

Exchange diets are the most commonly used because they are simple and require a minimum of calculation. The basic lists were compiled years ago in a joint effort of the American Diabetes Association, the American Dietetic Association, and the Chronic Disease Division of the United States Public Health Service. Many variations have evolved through the years, but all are basically similar. One variation is included here as Table 1.

Major foodstuffs have been categorized according to the amount of carbohydrate, protein, and fat they contain. It is wise to remember that the stated content represents an average value. Thus, when individual items are compared with food tables, there may be some discrepancy. These variations are minor and should be of no practical concern.

The following example illustrates use of the exchange system:

Prescription	Sample menu	Sample menu
2 meat exchanges	2 eggs	2 ounces Canadian bacon
1 bread exchange	1 slice toast	½ cup oatmeal with 2 tablespoons
1 fruit	½ cup orange juice	raisins
1 milk	1 cup milk	1 cup milk
1 fat	1 slice bacon	2 tablespoons light cream for cereal
		coffee

Generally your diet prescription will include a given number of meat, milk, fruit, vegetable, and bread exchanges. It should also include some suggestions for the distribution of these exchanges throughout the day, as this will influence their effect. It is beyond the scope of this book to teach the exchange system to previously uninstructed patients. If you have this kind of diet and do not clearly understand how to use it, request help from your physician or a consulting dietitian.

Note that one exchange does not necessarily equal one serving. When you consult your exchange list, always note the amount of food permitted for one exchange. Complete lists are included in Table 1, page 8.

Vegetables are divided into two general categories. Group A vegetables contain little carbohydrate, protein, or fat and if eaten raw may be used as desired. If cooked, 1 cup is allowed per exchange. Group B vegetables contain approximately 7 grams of carbohydrate, 2 grams of protein, and 35 calories in a ½ cup (1 exchange) serving.

A fruit exchange varies in amount depending upon the kind chosen. Each fruit exchange supplies 10 grams of carbohydrate and 40 calories.

Each bread exchange contains about 15 grams of carbohydrate, 2 grams of protein, and 70 calories. Note that cereals, crackers, beans, peas, potatoes, and similar foods are included with the bread exchanges. Portions vary.

Each meat exchange supplies approximately 7 grams of protein, 5 grams of fat, and 75 calories. Eggs, cheese, and peanut butter are included on this list. Portions, of course, vary.

One fat exchange supplies about 5 grams of fat and 45 calories. Butter, bacon, cream, salad dressings, nuts, olives, and avocados are included in this list because of their high fat content. No allowance is made for the carbohydrate and protein content of the nuts because small amounts are usually eaten. If you eat large amounts regularly, your dietitian or physician will need to adjust the remainder of your diet accordingly. The exact content of most nuts is included in Table 2, page 12.

Each milk exchange supplies approximately 12 grams of carbohydrate, 8 grams of protein, 10 grams of fat, and 170 calories. Note adjustment for skim milk in exchange lists.

In 1976 the exchange lists were revised. These revisions were made because of the concern for total caloric intake and the modification of fat intake currently being taught. Because many of you were taught your exchange diet prior to 1976, we have included both the revised and the old exchange lists. The differences are as follows for the revised version.

List 1 The milk exchanges are based on skim milk. You will need to omit fat exchanges from the regular allotment if you are using 2 percent or whole milk. You may simply use the old lists if you prefer.

List 2 Vegetable exchanges. Includes all vegetables except starchy ones. One half (½) cup is one exchange and averages 25 calories on the new system.

List 3 Fruit exchanges. Includes all fruits and fruit juices. It is presumed that no sugar has been added.

List 4 Bread exchanges. Includes bread, cereals, crackers, beans, starchy vegetables, and some prepared foods.

List 5 Meat exchanges. This is based on lean meats. One-half (½) fat exchange needs to be omitted for each exchange of medium fat meat. Omit 1 fat exchange for high fat meats.

List 6 Includes all fat exchanges. The foods in bold type are polyunsaturated. The regular type implies saturated fat.

You may simply find all of this unnecessarily confusing. If you were taught your diet before 1976, use the second set of tables. If taught after 1976, use the new tables. You will obtain the same results in either case.

WEIGHED DIET

This is the most demanding of all diabetic diets and is usually limited to those who must exercise maximum caution in the amount of carbohydrate they eat. Special instruction must be given to any patient who must use this kind of diet. A working knowledge of the exchange system will greatly simplify the adaptation to a weighed diet, but, in addition, one must purchase and know how to use a good food scale that weighs in grams. The gram is a very small unit of measure, roughly equal to 1/30th of an ounce. For example, there are 5 grams of fat in 1 teaspoonful, or 5 grams, of oil. Virtually all weighed diets use this system of measure. Properly used, the weighed diet can contribute significantly to good health in persons whose diabetes is hard to control. Many overweight persons with only mild diabetes would also do well to learn this system and use it until their weight approaches normal. The weighed diet actually permits the greatest flexibility in meal planning because the carbohydrate, protein, and fat content of each component is known. It is therefore possible to manipulate any recipe if the principles of the weighed diet are understood. This is its primary advantage.

Homemakers who enjoy creating and revising recipes will usually prefer the weighed-diet approach. These principles are simpler to apply to casseroles and other mixed dishes than are exchange principles.

Weighed diets are not simple, however, and individual instruction by a dietitian will be necessary. The principles outlined here will not suffice without additional instruction that takes individual problems into account.

Liquid food, such as milk, can generally be measured accurately in a standard measuring cup. Breads, meats, vegetables, and other foods must be weighed. Only the edible portion of food should be weighed.

Excess fat and bones should be removed from meat before weighing. Peelings and seeds should be removed from fruit. Food tables generally give values for cooked foods and note exceptions.

Your diet prescription will include the total grams of carbohydrate, protein, and fat permitted each day. A 1500-calorie-diet prescription might permit 150 grams of carbohydrate, 70 grams of protein, and 70 grams of fat for the entire day. A sample menu is shown below:

	C	P	F
2 eggs	0	14	10
1 slice toast (25 grams)	15	2	0
1 teaspoon margarine (5 grams)	0	0	5
1 cup of skim milk (240 grams)	12	8	0
Orange juice (100 grams)	10	0	0
	37	24	15

It must be emphasized here that 150 grams of carbohydrate does not mean 150 grams of food. It means a quantity of food that will supply 150 grams of carbohydrate. The same is, of course, true for protein and fat. Note in the example above that the slice of toast weighs 25 grams, but it supplies 15 grams of carbohydrate and 2 grams of protein for a total of 17 grams. The difference (25 minus 17) represents water and indigestible fibers. The carbohydrate, protein, and fat content of various foods can be determined from the food-content lists (Table 2).

Patients are rarely well enough instructed to use this system to its fullest potential. A good dietitian can be quite helpful to patients on such a program.

All diabetic diets share only one factor: They all require restriction of carbohydrate intake, especially sugar. Therefore, all foods that contain large amounts of carbohydrate, whether as sugar or as a starch, must be weighed or measured very carefully. The higher the carbohydrate content, the more carefully the food must be measured.

In my experience, the area of greatest insecurity for most newly diagnosed diabetics involves their diet. Many elderly diabetics eat the same boring menu over and over because they are hesitant to experiment with the exchange lists. This probably reflects a lack of understanding of basic principles. If you do not fully understand the diet recommended for you, and if your physician cannot take the time to explain it so that you do understand it, then seek help elsewhere. Large towns have an abundance of well-trained dietitians, many of whom do consulting work. Their fees are reasonable; they are expert in this field and are often good teachers. Each state has a chapter of the American Dietetic Association. The dietitian at your local hospital is probably a member and could perhaps direct you to someone who would help with your diet or could at least furnish the address of the American Dietetic Association. County and state health departments have well-trained nutritionists who will either help you themselves or recommend someone who will. The American Diabetes Association has branches in most states (see Appendix). These associations vary widely in the services they render, but many have consulting dietitians who are willing to give dietary help.

TABLE 1. UNREVISED EXCHANGE LISTS

These are the Unrevised Exchange Lists used with diets prescribed prior to 1976. If your diet was prescribed after 1976, use the "Revised Exchange Lists" on page 17.

In planning meals with diet exchanges, foods are divided into six groups. The foods in any one exchange group have approximately the same food values and may be substituted or exchanged for one another. The exchange groups and their food values are as follows:

Exchange list no.	Type	Amount	Weight (grams)	Content of one exchange (grams of carbohydrate, protein, fat; total calories)			
				C	P	F	Calories
1	Milk	1 cup	240	12	8	10	170
2A	Vegetable	½–1 cup	100		Minimal		
2B	Vegetable	½ cup	100	7	2		35
3	Fruit	1 serving	Varies	10			40
4	Bread	1 slice	25	15	2		70
5	Meat	1 ounce	30		7	5	75
6	Fat	1 teaspoon	5			5	45

LIST 1: MILK EXCHANGES

(Carbohydrate, 12 grams; protein, 8 grams; fat, 10 grams; calories, 170.)

	Measure	Grams
Buttermilk*	1 cup	240
Milk, evaporated*	½ cup	120
Milk, skim, powdered, instant*	⅓ cup	25

| Milk, skim* | 1 cup | 240 |
| Milk, whole | 1 cup | 240 |

*Two fat exchanges, or 85 calories, are "saved" if milk is "fat-free."

LIST 2A: VEGETABLE EXCHANGES

(Contain little carbohydrate, protein, or calories; often referred to as 3 percent vegetables, as that is approximate amount of carbohydrate they contain; need not be counted in amounts up to 1 cup, except tomatoes, which are limited to ½ cup.)

Asparagus	Greens:	Lettuce
Beans, string and wax	Beet Greens	Mushrooms
Broccoli	Chard, Swiss	Okra
Brussels sprouts	Collards	Parsley
Cabbage	Dandelion	Peppers
Cauliflower	Escarole	Radishes
Celery	Kale	Sauerkraut
Chicory	Mustard	Squash, summer
Chives	Romaine	Tomatoes or juice
Cucumbers	Spinach	Vegetable juice
Eggplant	Turnip greens	Water cress

LIST 2B: VEGETABLE EXCHANGES

(Carbohydrate, 7 grams; protein, 2 grams; calories, 35; often referred to as 7 percent vegetables, as that is approximate amount of carbohydrate they contain. One serving is ½ cup or 100 grams.)

Artichoke	Onions	Squash, winter
Beets	Peas, green	Tomato purée, canned
Carrots or juice	Pumpkin	Turnips
Celery root	Rutabagas	Vegetables, frozen, mixed
Kohlrabi	Salsify (oyster plant)	

LIST 3: FRUIT EXCHANGES

(Carbohydrate, 10 grams; calories, 40.)

	Measure	Grams
Apple	½ medium	75
Apple juice	⅓ cup	80
Applesauce	½ cup	100
Apricots, dried	4 halves	20
Apricots, fresh or canned	2 medium	100
Banana	½ small	50
Berries (strawberries, raspberries, blackberries)	¾ cup	100

Blueberries	½ cup	65
Cantaloupe (6 inches in diameter)	¼	200
Cherries	10 large	65
Dates	2	15
Figs, dried	1 small	15
Figs, fresh	2 large	50
Fruit cocktail, canned	½ cup	100
Grapefruit	½ small	100
Grapefruit juice	½ cup	100
Grape juice	¼ cup	60
Grapes	12 large	65
Honeydew melon (7 inches in diameter)	⅛	200
Mango	½ small	65
Nectarine	1 small	60
Orange	1 small	100
Orange juice	½ cup	100
Papaya	⅓ medium	100
Peach	1 medium (½ cup)	100
Pear	1 small (½ cup)	100
Pineapple	½ cup	80
Pineapple juice	⅓ cup	80
Plums	2 small	100
Prune juice	¼ cup	60
Prunes, dried	2 medium	25
Raisins	2 tablespoons	15
Tangerine	1 large	100
Watermelon	1 cup	200

LIST 4: BREAD EXCHANGES

(Carbohydrate, 15 grams; protein, 2 grams; calories, 70.)

	Measure	Grams
Bread	1 slice	25
Biscuit (2 inches in diameter)	1	35
Bread sticks	4 4-inch pieces	20
Cornbread (1½-inch cube)	1	35
Hamburger bun	½	25
Melba toast	4 pieces	20
Muffin (2 inches in diameter)	1	35
Roll (plain)	1 medium	25
Cereals, cooked	½ cup	100
Dry, flake, and puff types	¾ cup	20
Crackers*		
Graham	3 square	20
Oyster	½ cup	20
Ry-Krisp	3 pieces	20
Saltines (2 inches square)	6	20

Soda (2½ inches square)	3	20
Zwieback	3	20
Flour	2½ tablespoons	20
Macaroni, rice, spaghetti, noodles (cooked)	½ cup	100
Popcorn	1 cup	15
Pretzels (toasted three-ring)	6	20
Vegetables		
Beans and peas, dried, cooked	½ cup	90
Corn	⅓ cup	80
Parsnips	½ cup	100
Potatoes, sweet, or yams	¼ cup	50
Potatoes, white	½ cup	100

*Crackers (except Ry-Krisp) are nutritionally very poor and should therefore be used rarely.

LIST 5: MEAT EXCHANGES

(Protein, 7 grams; fat, 5 grams; calories, 75. Note that all items are given in cooked portion.)

	Measure	Grams
Cheese (any except cottage and cream)	1 ounce	30
Cheese, cottage	¼ cup	45
Egg	1	
Fish (canned tuna, salmon)	¼ cup	30
Fish (salmon, cod, trout, halibut)	1 ounce	30
Lunch meat (4½ by ⅛ inches)	1 slice	45
Meat and poultry (beef, lamb, pork, liver, chicken, etc.)	1 ounce	30
Peanut butter (omit ½ fruit exchange and 2 fat exchanges)	2 tablespoons	30
Shellfish (crab, lobster)	¼ cup	45
Shellfish (shrimp, clams, oysters)	5 medium	45
Wiener (8 or 9 per pound)	1	50

LIST 6: FAT EXCHANGES

(Fat, 5 grams; calories, 45. Those that appear in bold type are low in cholesterol.)

	Measure	Grams
Avocado (4 inches in diameter)	⅛	25
Bacon, crisp	1 slice	10
Butter or **margarine**	1 teaspoon	5
Cream, heavy (40 percent)	1 tablespoon	15
Cream, light (20 percent)	2 tablespoons	30
Cream cheese	1 tablespoon	15
French dressing	1 tablespoon	15
Mayonnaise	1 teaspoon	5

Nuts	6 small	10
Oil, vegetable	1 teaspoon	5
Olives	5 small	30

TABLE 2. FOOD-CONTENT LISTS
(in gram weights)

MILK*

	Weight (grams)	C	P	F	Calories
Buttermilk	240	12	8		85
Milk, evaporated	120	12	8	10	170
Milk, evaporated, skim	120	12	8		85
Milk, powdered, instant	25	12	8	10	170
Milk, powdered, instant skim	25	12	8		85
Milk, skim	240	12	8		85
Milk, whole	240	12	8	10	170
Yogurt, plain†	240	12	8	4	120

*If you use 2 percent milk, call your dairy to obtain the analysis. This milk sometimes contains 2 percent additional milk solids in addition to a lowered fat content of 2 percent.

†The fat content of yogurt varies.

VEGETABLES

Group A: 3 percent carbohydrate

(Average 3 grams of carbohydrate and 15 calories in 100-gram serving.)

Asparagus	Greens:	Mushrooms
Beans, string and wax	Beet greens	Okra
Broccoli	Chard, Swiss	Parsley
Brussels sprouts	Collards	Pepper
Cabbage	Dandelion	Radishes
Cauliflower	Escarole	Sauerkraut
Celery	Kale	Squash, summer
Chicory	Mustard	Tomatoes or juice
Chives	Romaine	Vegetable juice
Cucumbers	Spinach	Water cress
Eggplant	Turnip greens	

Group B: 7 percent carbohydrate

(Average 7 grams of carbohydrate, 2 grams of protein, and 35 calories in 100-gram serving.)

Artichoke	Onions	Squash, winter
Beets	Peas, green	Tomato purée, canned
Carrots or juice	Pumpkin	Turnips
Celery root	Rutabagas	Vegetables, frozen mixed
Kohlrabi	Salsify (oyster plant)	

MISCELLANEOUS VEGETABLES

(Values given are for cooked weight.)

	Weight (grams)	C	P	F	Calories
Beans, lima (fresh or frozen)	90	15	2		70
Beans or peas, dried	90	15	2		70
Corn	80	15	2		70
Parsnips	100	15	2		70
Potatoes, sweet, or yams	50	15	2		70
Soybeans	100	9	10	5	120

FRUITS

(Values given are for edible portion—fresh, cooked, canned, or frozen without sugar.)

Group A: 5 percent carbohydrate

(100 grams will average 5 grams of carbohydrate and 20 calories.)

Cantaloupe	Rhubarb
Honeydew melon	Watermelon
Lemons or juice	

Group B: 10 percent carbohydrate

(100 grams will average 10 grams of carbohydrate and 40 calories.)

Applesauce	Loganberries
Apricots	Oranges or juice
Blackberries or juice	Papayas
Boysenberries	Peaches
Cranberries	Pears
Currants	Plums
Fruit cocktail (canned)	Raspberries
Grapefruit or juice	Strawberries
Huckleberries	Tangerines
Limes or juice	

Group C: 15 percent carbohydrate

(100 grams will average 15 grams of carbohydrate and 60 calories.)

Apples or juice	Nectarines
Blueberries	Persimmons
Cherries	Pineapple or juice
Grapes or juice	Pomegranates
Mangoes	

Group D: 20 percent carbohydrate

(100 grams will average 20 grams of carbohydrate and 80 calories.)

Bananas
Figs
Prune juice

MISCELLANEOUS FRUITS

	Weight (grams)	C	P	F	Calories
Apricots, dried	20	10			40
Avocado	100	5	2	15	165
Cranberry juice, dietetic	100	2			11
Dates, dried figs, raisins	15	10			40
Prunes, dried (seed weight included)	25	10			40

BREADS AND CEREALS

	Weight (grams)	C	P	F	Calories
Bread					
Biscuit	35	15	2	6	125
Bread sticks, melba toast	20	15	2		70
Corn bread	35	15	2	3	100
Hamburger bun	55	30	4		140
Muffin (2 inches in diameter)	35	15	2	3	100
White, whole-wheat, rye, plain rolls	25	15	2		70
Cereals					
Cereals, cooked	100	15	2		70
Cereals, uncooked, dry weight	20	15	2		70
Cereals, packaged, ready-to-eat	20	15	2		70
Cornstarch	8	7			30
Wheat germ	10	5	3	1	35

Crackers
  Graham, oyster, Ry-krisp,
    saltines, soda, zwieback   20   15   3   1   35

Flour
  Rye and wheat   10   7   1   35
  Soy*   10   3   5   1   40

Macaroni, noodles, rice,
  spaghetti (cooked weight)   100   15   2   70

*The analysis of soy flour varies considerably among milling companies.

MEAT, POULTRY, FISH, CHEESE, EGGS

	Weight (grams)	C	P	F	Calories
Beef, lamb, pork, ham	30		7	5	75
Cheese					
American, Swiss	30		7	9	110
Cottage	45		7	3	55
Eggs					
Whole	1		7	5	75
White	1		3		15
Yolk	1		4	5	60
Fish (salmon, cod, trout, halibut)	30		7	1	40
Lunch meat	45		5	8	90
Peanut butter	30	6	8	14	180
Poultry, dried beef, veal, game, liver	30		7	3	55
Shellfish (crab, lobster, shrimp, clams, oysters)	45		7	1	40
Wiener	50		7	10	125

FATS

	Weight (grams)	C	P	F	Calories
Bacon, crisp	10		2	5	55
Butter or margarine	5			4	35
Cream, heavy (40 percent)	15			6	55
Cream, light (20 percent)	30	1	1	6	65
Cream cheese	15		1	6	55
French dressing	15	2		6	60
Mayonnaise	5			4	35
Neufchâtel cheese	30	1	3	7	70
Nuts, average for all nuts*	10	2	2	6	70
Almonds	10	2	2	5	60
Beechnuts	10	2	2	5	60
Brazil nuts	10	1	1	7	70

Butternuts	10	1	2	6	65
Cashews	10	3	2	5	65
Filberts	10	2	1	6	65
Hickory nuts	10	1	1	7	70
Macadamia nuts	10	2	1	7	75
Peanuts	10	2	3	5	65
Pecans	10	2	1	7	75
Walnuts, English	10	2	2	6	65
Oil, vegetable	5			5	45
Olives, green (seed weight included)	50			6	55
Olives, ripe (seed weight included)	30			6	55

*Unless larger quantities of specific nuts are desired, use the "average" figure for nuts.

MISCELLANEOUS FOODS

	Weight (grams)	C	P	F	Calories
Carbonated beverage (sweet)*	100	10			40
Catsup or chili sauce	15	4			15
Cocoa, unsweetened	5	1		1	15
Ovaltine	10	7	1		30
Ice cream, dietetic or sugar-free	50	10	2	5	95
Ice cream, plain, vanilla	50	10	2	6	100
Popcorn, popped	15	12	2		55
Potato chips and Fritos	15	7	1	6	85
Soy sauce	30	3			15
Sunflower seeds	15	3	4	7	90
Yeast, brewer's, powder	10	4	4		30

*Use sugar-sweetened carbonated beverages only in emergencies, such as illness or insulin reactions.

FREE FOODS

(The following items have negligible carbohydrate, protein, and fat, and may be used as desired.)

Artificial sweeteners	Mustard
Broth and bouillon (fat free)	Pepper, other spices and herbs
Coffee	Pickles, unsweetened
Flavoring extracts (vanilla, lemon, etc.)	Rennet tablets (junket)
Gelatin, unsweetened	Tea
Gelatin dessert mix, sugarless	Vinegar

The figures used for determining these tables were taken from *Composition of Foods, U.S. Department of Agriculture Handbook No. 8* (Washington, D.C.: G.P.O., 1963), and Charles F. Church, *Food Values of Portions Commonly Used* (Philadelphia: J. B. Lippincott Co., 1966).

TABLE 3. 1976 REVISED EXCHANGE LISTS

These are the 1976 Revised Exchange Lists. Use these tables if you were taught your diet since 1976. If you were instructed prior to 1976, use the set of Exchange Lists beginning on page 8.

LIST 1: MILK EXCHANGES

One exchange of milk contains: carbohydrate, 12 g; protein, 8 g, fat, trace (80 calories).

This list shows the kinds and amounts of milk products to use for one milk exchange. Those that appear in bold type are nonfat. Low-fat and whole milk contain saturated fat.

Nonfat Fortified Milk

Skim or nonfat milk	1 cup
Powdered (nonfat dry, before adding liquid)	⅓ cup
Canned, evaporated—skim	½ cup
Buttermilk from skim milk	1 cup
Yogurt made from skim milk (plain, unflavored)	1 cup

Low-fat Fortified Milk

1% fat fortified milk (omit ½ fat exchange)	1 cup
2% fat fortified milk (omit 1 fat exchange)	1 cup
Yogurt made from 2% fortified milk (plain unflavored) (omit 1 fat exchange)	1 cup

Whole Milk

Whole milk (omit 2 fat exchanges)	1 cup
Canned, evaporated whole milk (omit 2 fat exchanges)	½ cup
Buttermilk made from whole milk (omit 2 fat exchanges)	1 cup
Yogurt made from whole milk (plain, unflavored) (omit 2 fat exchanges)	1 cup

LIST 2: VEGETABLE EXCHANGES

One exchange of vegetable contains: carbohydrate, 5 g, protein, 2 g (25 calories).

This list shows the kinds of vegetables to use for one vegetable exchange. One exchange is ½ cup.

Asparagus
Bean sprouts
Beets
Broccoli
Brussels sprouts

Greens:
Mustard
Spinach
Turnip
Mushrooms

Cabbage	Okra
Carrots	Onions
Cauliflower	Rhubarb
Celery	Rutabaga
Cucumbers	Sauerkraut
Eggplant	String beans, green or yellow
Greens:	Summer squash
Beet	Tomatoes
Chard	Tomato juice
Collard	Turnips
Dandelion	Vegetable juice
Kale	Zucchini

The following raw vegetables may be used as desired:

Chicory	Lettuce
Chinese cabbage	Parsley
Endive	Radishes
Escarole	Water cress

Starchy vegetables are found in the bread exchange list.

LIST 3: FRUIT EXCHANGES

One exchange of fruit contains: carbohydrate, 10 g (40 calories).
    This list shows the kinds and amounts of fruits to use for one fruit exchange.

Apple	1 small	Mango	½ small
Apple juice	⅓ cup	Melon:	
Applesauce		Cantaloupe	¼ small
(unsweetened)	½ cup	Honeydew	⅛ medium
Apricots, fresh	2 medium	Watermelon	1 cup
Apricots, dried	4 halves	Nectarine	1 small
Banana	½ small	Orange	1 small
Berries:		Orange juice	½ cup
Blackberries	½ cup	Papaya	¾ cup
Blueberries	½ cup	Peach	1 medium
Raspberries	½ cup	Pear	1 small
Strawberries	¾ cup	Persimmon, native	1 medium
Cherries	10 large	Pineapple	½ cup
Cider	⅓ cup	Pineapple juice	⅓ cup
Dates	2	Plums	2 medium
Figs, dried	1	Prune juice	¼ cup
Figs, fresh	1	Prunes	2 medium
Grapefruit	½	Raisins	2 tablespoons
Grapefruit juice	½ cup	Tangerine	1 medium
Grape juice	¼ cup		
Grapes	12		

Cranberries may be used as desired if no sugar is added.

LIST 4: BREAD EXCHANGES

One exchange of bread contains: carbohydrate, 15 g, protein, 2 g (70 calories).

This list shows the kinds and amounts of breads, cereals, starchy vegetables, and prepared foods to use for one bread exchange.

Bread

Bagel, small	½
Dried crumbs, bread	3 tablespoons
English muffin, small	½
Frankfurter roll	½
Hamburger roll	½
Raisin	1 slice
Roll, plain bread	1
Rye or pumpernickel	1 slice
Tortilla, 6 inch	1
White (including French and Italian)	1 slice
Whole-wheat	1 slice

Starchy vegetables

Corn	⅓ cup
Corn on the cob	1 small
Lima beans	½ cup
Parsnips	⅔ cup
Peas, green (canned or frozen)	½ cup
Potato, white	1 small
Potato (mashed)	½ cup
Potato, sweet, or yam	¼ cup
Pumpkin	¾ cup
Squash, acorn or butternut	½ cup

Cereal

Bran flakes	½ cup
Cereal (cooked)	½ cup
Cornmeal (dry)	2 tablespoons
Grits (cooked)	½ cup
Flour	2½ tablespoons
Other ready-to-eat (unsweetened) cereal	¾ cup
Pasta (cooked)	
(spaghetti, noodles, macaroni)	½ cup
Popcorn (popped, no fat added)	3 cups
Puffed cereal (unfrosted)	1 cup
Rice or barley (cooked)	½ cup
Wheat germ	¼ cup

Crackers

Arrowroot	3
Graham, 2½-inch square	2

Matzo, 4 inch × 6 inch	½
Oyster	20
Pretzels, 3⅛ inches long × ⅛ inch diameter	25
Rye wafers, 2 inches × 3½ inches	3
Saltines	6
Soda, 2½-inch square	4

Dried peas, beans and lentils

Beans, peas, lentils (dried and cooked)	½ cup
Baked beans, no pork (canned)	¼ cup

Prepared Foods

Biscuit, 2-inch diameter	1
(omit 1 fat exchange)	
Corn bread, 2 inches × 2 inches × 1 inch	1
(omit 1 fat exchange)	
Corn muffin (2-inch diameter)	1
(omit 1 fat exchange)	
Crackers, round butter type	5
(omit 1 fat exchange)	
Muffin, plain small	1
(omit 1 fat exchange)	
Potatoes, French-fried,	8
(length 2 inches to 3½ inches)	
(omit 1 fat exchange)	
Potato or corn chips	15
(omit 2 fat exchanges)	
Pancake, 5 inch × ½ inch	1
(omit 1 fat exchange)	
Waffle, 5 inch × ½ inch	1
(omit 1 fat exchange)	

LIST 5: MEAT EXCHANGES

Low-fat meat

One exchange of low-fat meat contains: protein, 7 grams; fat, 3 grams (55 calories). This list shows the kinds and amounts of lean meat and other protein-rich foods to use for one low-fat meat exchange.

Beef: baby beef (very lean), chipped beef, chuck, flank steak, plate ribs, plate skirt steak, round (bottom, top), rump (all cuts), spare ribs, tenderloin, tripe	1 ounce
Cheeses: containing less than 5% butterfat	1 ounce
Cottage cheese, dry and 2% butterfat	¼ cup
Dried beans and peas (omit 1 bread exchange)	½ cup
Fish:	
Any fresh or frozen	1 ounce
Canned crab, lobster, mackerel, salmon, or tuna	¼ cup

Clams, oysters, scallops, shrimp	5, or ounce
Sardines, drained	3
Lamb: leg, loin (roast and chops), rib, shank, shoulder, sirloin	1 ounce
Pork: ham, leg (whole rump, center shank), smoked center slices	1 ounce
Poultry: chicken (meat without skin), Cornish game hen, guinea hen, pheasant, turkey	1 ounce
Veal: cutlets, leg, loin, rib, shank, shoulder	1 ounce

Medium-fat Meat

For each exchange of medium-fat meat, omit ½ fat exchange.

Beef: corned beef (canned), ground (15% fat), rib eye, round (ground commercial)	1 ounce
Cheese:	
Farmer's cheese, mozzarella, Neufchâtel, ricotta	1 ounce
Parmesan	3 tablespoons
Cottage cheese, creamed	¼ cup
Egg (high in cholesterol)	1
Liver, heart, kidney, and sweetbreads (these are high in cholesterol)	1 ounce
Peanut butter (omit 2 additional fat exchanges)	2 tablespoons
Pork: boiled ham, Boston butt, Canadian bacon, loin (all cuts), tenderloin, shoulder arm (picnic), shoulder blade	1 ounce

High-fat Meat

For each exchange of high-fat meat, omit 1 fat exchange.

Beef: brisket, chuck (ground commercial), corned beef (brisket), ground beef (more than 20% fat), hamburger (commercial), roasts (rib), steaks (club, rib)	1 ounce
Cheese: Cheddar types	1 ounce
Cold cuts, 4½ inches square × ⅛ inch	1 slice
Pork: country-style ham, deviled ham, ground pork, loin (back ribs), spare ribs	1 ounce
Poultry: capon, duck (domestic), goose	1 ounce
Veal: breast	1 ounce
Wiener	1 small

LIST 6: FAT EXCHANGES

One exchange of fat contains: fat, 5 grams (45 calories). This list shows the kinds and amounts of fat-containing foods for 1 fat exchange. To plan a diet low in saturated fat, select only those exchanges that appear in bold type—they are polyunsaturated.

Avocado, 4 inches in diameter	⅛
Bacon, crisp	1 strip
Bacon fat	1 teaspoon
Butter	1 teaspoon
Cream, heavy	1 tablespoon
Cream, light	2 tablespoons
Cream, sour	2 tablespoons
Cream cheese	1 tablespoon
French dressing‡	1 tablespoon
Italian dressing‡	1 tablespoon
Lard	1 teaspoon
Margarine, regular stick	1 teaspoon
Margarine, soft, tub or stick	1 teaspoon
Mayonnaise‡	1 teaspoon
Nuts:	
Almonds	10 whole
Pecans†	2 large whole
Peanuts, Spanish†	20 whole
Peanuts, Virginia†	10 whole
Walnuts	6 small
Other†	6 small
Oil: corn, cottonseed, safflower, soy, or sunflower	1 teaspoon
Oil, olive†	1 teaspoon
Oil, peanut†	1 teaspoon
Olives†	5 small
Salad dressing, mayonnaise type‡	2 teaspoons
Salt pork	¾-inch cube

†Fat content is ordinarily monounsaturated.

‡If made with corn, cottonseed, safflower, soy or sunflower oil, can be used on fat-modified diet.

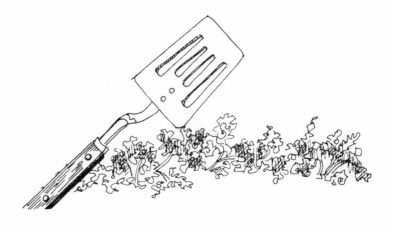

CHAPTER 2

General Nutritional
Principles

All foods are composed of protein, carbohydrate, and fat, either alone or in combination. Each of these components serves a unique function in the body, and they are only slightly interchangeable. Calories are present in all of these components of food. Calories are simply units of energy and are present in varying amounts in almost everything we eat.

A gram of carbohydrate will contain 4 calories;
          an ounce about 112.
A gram of protein will contain 4 calories;
          an ounce about 112.
A gram of fat will contain 9 calories;
          an ounce 227 calories.

An easy conclusion here is that the elimination of fat from one's diet would be twice as productive in reducing calories as eliminating either carbohydrate or protein. While that is true, it does not take into account the fact that all foods, and therefore nutrients, are utilized in a more beneficial manner in the presence of some fat. Fat serves the useful function of slowing digestion and delaying the onset of hunger. Certainly excess fat can be eliminated, but if the aim is just to reduce calories, they should be eliminated from both carbohydrate and fat allotments. Protein is rarely taken in excess quantity and should not be reduced in order to reduce calories.

CARBOHYDRATE

Carbohydrate includes both starch and sugar. The carbohydrate in our diet is used by the body for energy. People who do heavy work or are active in athletics will need more than the sedentary office worker. If more carbohydrate is eaten than is expended in energy, it will be converted into fat and stored in the body for future use. If these stores are not used periodically, more and more fat will be accumulated and obesity will result. It is of some importance to determine whether your weight is stable so proper adjustment in your food intake can be made. Even a hundred excess calories a day will make a difference of about 10 pounds in a year. Weigh regularly on a reliable set of scales. Try to weigh at the same time of day and with similar, or no, clothes. If your weight is varying in the same direction—for example, going up continuously—look over your diet and omit one of the energy sources until you are again at a reasonable weight.

Juvenile diabetics often have the opposite problem of being unable to maintain their body weight. This most often is the result of uncontrolled diabetes, but it can also be because the prescribed diet may not include enough calories.

If you are losing weight, your doctor will want to know.

Sources of starch include such diverse things as potatoes, fruit, beans, and bread. Most vegetables contain some starch. All fruits contain carbohydrate as both starch and sugar. That it is "natural" sugar doesn't matter a whit as far as calories are concerned. Fruits are delicious and nutritious, but they must be recognized as common sources of excess carbohydrate.

A daily requirement of carbohydrate must be determined individually, since it depends so greatly on activity and age. Insulin-dependent diabetics should not decrease their carbohydrate below 100 grams, because some degree of ketosis will result. All diabetics should receive professional guidance before undertaking a weight-reduction program. There are many reducing diets in circulation that are entirely unsuitable for diabetic patients. Never try diets from newspapers or magazines without your doctor's approval. All forms of carbohydrate, whether sugar or starch, contain about 4 calories per gram, or 112 calories per ounce.

PROTEIN

Proteins are composed of fragments known as amino acids. There are twenty-two amino acids, which combine in a variety of ways to constitute the protein we eat. Of these twenty-two amino acids, all except eight can be produced in the body, provided other dietary intake is adequate. These eight essential acids must be ingested daily to maintain health.

Protein is used in the body to repair vital structures such as bone, hair, skin, muscle, and blood in the adult, and to permit formation of these tissues in the growing child. Generous amounts of protein should be taken by both children and adults.

Unfortunately, proteins are usually expensive, and, consequently, inadequate amounts may be eaten in low-income situations. There are several relatively inexpensive sources of good-quality protein, of which powdered milk and soybeans are outstanding examples. A quart of powdered milk costs about 25 cents in today's market and furnishes about half the daily protein requirement for adults and children. Soybeans are about equivalent to meat in protein content and provide most of the protein in vegetarian diets. The person who shops and cooks bears a significant responsibility to learn relative protein values so that all members of the family may be intelligently fed.

Protein is especially important as a source of calories for the diabetic, since it causes minimal change in the blood sugar and may act as a stabilizer for carbohydrate taken along with it. Protein requires more digestion prior to absorption into the bloodstream, and, therefore, provides only small amounts of calories over several hours.

During the past few years, a large community of young vegetarians has emerged. This is partly for religious or ethical reasons and partly because of concern for worldwide protein shortages. Unfortunately, few of these young converts have had reliable advice about quantities of foods necessary to provide adequate protein for good health. There has been a wealth of misinformation about sources of protein and little discussion of varying quality of the different proteins. It is certainly possible to be well nourished as a vegetarian, but you must have a very clear understanding of where protein occurs and make a determined effort to obtain it at every opportunity. The Seventh Day Adventist churches have taught courses to their parishioners for years that would be of great benefit to anyone trying to eat by vegetarian principles.

Meat, milk, cheese, and eggs are the most common sources of protein in the nonvegetarian's diet. Nuts, beans and soy products can be combined with grains and other vegetables to provide protein for the vegetarian. Although low protein intake is entirely compatible with life, it is not necessarily compatible with good health.

All proteins contain about 4 calories per gram, or 112 calories per ounce.

FAT

Most people do not think of fat as a nutrient, yet fats contain essential fatty acids necessary for good health. Public attitudes toward fat have undergone a remarkable change over the last decade. Although the cholesterol debate has raged for more than a quarter of a century, it remains a debate. The American Heart Association has made a determined effort to change the eating habits of all Americans to include less saturated fat and more unsaturated fat.

As an early convert to that philosophy, I confess to being less impressed by its virtues at this time in my life than I was as a young physician. Certainly there are some patients who must limit their intake of cholesterol, but most people handle dietary cholesterol (that is to say cholesterol present in foods) quite normally. There is a larger group of people that should simply restrict calories, and many of these calories will logically be in the fat category. Everyone needs some saturated fat, but no one is sure exactly how much.

Every diabetic patient should be under the care of a physician, and it is most likely that cholesterol and triglyceride levels will be measured at regular intervals. You pay your doctor to give you advice about things you don't understand. Often there are things that no one understands completely, but your own doctor is the person best equipped to advise you what to do about your dietary fat. If your doctor has advised you to cut down your cholesterol intake, then try to learn what is saturated and what is unsaturated fat. If you use vegetable oils, nuts, and other seeds, you will get some unsaturated fat. If you eat meat, cheese, and eggs, you will get saturated fat. The amount you will need is dependent upon your age, exercise levels, and whether you must take insulin.

One of the good things fat does is to slow down the rate of digestion. This permits the food taken at meals to last several hours instead of a few minutes. That's a great addition to the program, especially if you take insulin injections. If your doctor has recommended that you increase the ratio of unsaturated fats to saturated fats, you will need to alter your choice of foods to accommodate that recommendation. All vegetable oils contain the essential fatty acids required for health. For this reason alone, your diet should contain a portion of unsaturated fat.

MINERALS

Minerals contain such diverse elements as iron, calcium, iodine, and cobalt. These are found in conjunction with carbohydrate and protein foods and are a necessary part of the diet of diabetics and nondiabetics alike.

There are wide differences in the daily requirements for minerals and trace elements among age groups and sexes. Growing children and women of childbearing age require more iron than do adult men and aged women. Growing children and pregnant women will require more calcium, among other things. Definite requirements for most of the essential trace elements are not known. It is mechanically difficult to determine these requirements, and about all that can be said with certainty is that "some" is needed for health. Even for well-studied minerals—such as calcium, phosphorus, and iron—discussions of minimum daily requirements still stir debate in learned circles. The National Research Council on Food and Nutrition periodically issues recommended levels of intake for all known essential foodstuffs, and their recommendations represent the best advice we have at the present time. These recommendations are usually given wide publicity, so it is easy to update your knowledge as we learn more and more about nutritional requirements.

CALCIUM

Calcium is necessary for strong healthy bones and teeth. It is also necessary for normal muscle function and is present at all times in the bloodstream. When enough calcium is not taken in the diet to supply these immediate needs, it will be dissolved out of the stores kept in the bones and teeth. Thus, if a diet deficient in calcium is followed for many years, the bones will gradually become depleted and may weaken.

Dairy products constitute the commonest source in the American diet. In fact, it is almost impossible to obtain the daily requirement if you don't use dairy products. Remember that skim milk and buttermilk contain the calcium without the saturated fat of whole milk. Don't cut out milk just because you need to eliminate fat. Cow's milk contains about 250 milligrams of calcium per cup. Small amounts of calcium are present in various vegetables, but because of other chemicals combined with it, these sources cannot be relied on for dietary needs. The recommended daily allowance for adults is 800 milligrams (that's three glasses of milk a day), and 1200 milligrams a day for pregnant or lactating women.

PHOSPHORUS

Phosphorus is calcium's teammate. Like calcium, it is also necessary for the calcification of bones and teeth. Phosphorus serves an additional function in controlling the release of energy from the oxidation or burning of carbohydrates, fat, and protein in the body. The recommended allowance is the same as for calcium, but the sources of phosphorus are more widespread and it is better absorbed. Avoid taking too much phosphorus; excessive intake of phosphorus will interfere with calcium absorption and deposition in bone.

It should be noted in this regard that carbonated beverages may contain up to 500 milligrams per can. Even "diet pops" have this shortcoming. Daily intake of these drinks is strongly discouraged. Phosphorus is found in dairy products, meat, eggs, cereals, and vegetables.

SODIUM

Sodium is part of the molecule of ordinary table salt. It is necessary for the maintenance of body fluids in normal amounts. Only in conditions of excessive heat and sweating is too little table salt a problem. Many patients who suffer from high blood pressure will be advised to limit their salt intake to 1 or 2 grams daily—the average American intake is about 5 grams daily.

Sodium occurs naturally in meats, milk, and vegetables. Table salt contains about 2 grams per teaspoon.

POTASSIUM

Potassium is present in all cells of the body and is necessary for the normal function of the muscles. It is also present in small amounts in a wide variety of foodstuffs. About 50 milligrams a day are required by healthy adults. Either too much or too little can cause a serious medical problem.

Potassium intake becomes a problem when diuretics ("water pills") are taken for high blood pressure or some other disease. These medications cause the body to lose more than the normal amount of potassium, and severe deficiency can occur. Never take such medications without your doctor's knowledge. Milk, fruit, nuts, and vegetables contain small amounts. If vegetables are cooked, much of the potassium will be lost in the cooking water, so it should be used along with the vegetable. We frequently make a broth from the vegetable cooking water. It makes a delicious dinner drink. But then it often is not possible to use dietary sources alone for replacement when medication is required and a supplement must be taken.

MAGNESIUM

Magnesium is needed in several enzyme systems in the body and is combined with calcium and phosphorus in bone. Soft tissue and all body fluids contain small amounts. Leafy green vegetables are good sources. The recommended daily allowance is 350 milligrams for men, 300 milligrams for women, and 450 milligrams for pregnant or lactating women.

IRON

Iron is necessary for normal blood formation. It is widespread in nature but is, unfortunately, difficult to absorb. Only about 10 percent of the iron present in vegetable sources will be absorbed even when a deficiency exists. About 20 percent of the iron present in meat will be absorbed.

A recent survey by the Department of Agriculture found that a very high percentage of young women were iron-deficient. Teenage girls are the commonest victims of iron deficiency. Their food intake is often irregular and of poor quality. In addition, they lose iron regularly through menstrual bleeding. An iron supplement is a sensible precaution for teenage girls.

Vegetarians may require a supplement even if they have no regular iron losses, since iron from vegetable sources is so poorly absorbed. Red meat and eggs are good sources.

The recommended allowance for postmenopausal women and for men is 10 milligrams daily. Menstruating and pregnant women should have at least 18 milligrams.

ZINC

Zinc has only recently been added to the list of essential nutrients. It is used in the body in numerous enzyme systems, is an integral part of the insulin molecule, and is necessary for good wound healing. The recommended daily allowance for adults is 15 milligrams. It is found in meat and leafy green vegetables.

IODINE

Iodine is necessary for normal thyroid function. Iodized salt is the most reliable source of iodine. It also occurs naturally in a variety of meats, seafoods, and vegetables. Many areas of the country are iodine-deficient zones. The soil in these areas does not contain iodine, and therefore food grown in these areas will not contain the expected amount. Recognition of this fact led many years ago to the addition of iodine to table salt. If iodized salt is used regularly, it will provide adequate iodine even in deficient zones.

Normal adults require about 60 micrograms per day.

VITAMINS

Vitamins, like trace minerals, are needed in small amounts for the maintenance of good health in diabetics and nondiabetics alike. Because vitamins occur naturally in association with varying amounts of protein, carbohydrate, and fat, the diabetic must be somewhat more sure of his sources than the nondiabetic. A person who can eat as much as he likes of the entire spectrum of foods should not suffer from vitamin deficiency. This, unhappily, is not the case with diabetics or many nondiabetics. Not only is the range of foods limited, but also the amount. It is, therefore, mandatory that all calories taken, especially as carbohydrate and fat, carry their full weight of vitamin content. This is especially important if calories are limited to less than 1500 a day.

There are two general categories of vitamins: those that dissolve in water and thus must be taken daily, and those that dissolve in fat and can be stored by the body for long periods of time. The water-soluble group includes all the B vitamins and vitamin C. If the diabetic is not well controlled, many of the water-soluble vitamins will be lost in the urine. The fat-soluble group includes vitamins A, D, E, and K.

VITAMIN A

Vitamin A is used in the body for maintenance of healthy eyes, skin, hair, and nails. Diabetics have more infections that involve the skin and nails than nondiabetics, and therefore all precautions should be taken to ensure the health of these tissues. Vitamin A is found in leafy green vegetables, yellow fruits and vegetables, and liver from all animals. Your diabetic diet's selection of fruit and vegetables provides for adequate vitamin A. This vitamin dissolves in fat but not in water. Therefore, it is stored in the body for long periods of time, and if taken one day and not used it may be saved for another day when the intake is not adequate. This is in contrast to the B and C vitamins, which are lost in the urine if not needed immediately by the body. About 5000 units of vitamin A are needed daily. This amount is present in one healthy carrot or ⅓ cup of cooked leafy green vegetable, such as turnip greens or spinach.

It is possible to take too much vitamin A, and therefore, good dietary sources are preferable to concentrated forms such as vitamin tablets.

When the National Research Council's recommended daily allowances were revised in 1974, they adopted the term "retinal equivalents" (RE) to be used instead of the units we are accustomed to using. The above stated 5000 units is equivalent to 1000 retinal equivalents.

VITAMIN D

The primary function of vitamin D is the building and maintenance of strong, healthy bones. It accomplishes this by influencing calcium and phosphorus absorption and is required by both children and adults.

About 400 units are needed daily, and fortified milk is the most reliable source, with 1 quart providing a day's allowance of 400 units. Keep in mind that skim milk may not be fortified with vitamin D. If skim milk is used exclusively and there is limited exposure to sunlight, it is sometimes necessary to provide a supplement, especially for growing children. Vitamin D is found in small amounts in liver and egg yolks, but these foods alone cannot supply the needed amount in most diets. Sunlight will convert some substances on skin into vitamin D. In warm areas where sunbathing is common, this contributes significantly to vitamin D needs.

Like vitamin A, vitamin D may be stored in the body for many days after it is taken. Too large a quantity may cause serious illness, and this complication is usually seen among people who take large amounts regularly by capsule. Again, it is better to rely upon a well-planned diet than upon vitamin supplements. Vitamin D should not be taken as a supplement unless specifically prescribed.

VITAMIN E

Vitamin E is one of the more recently discovered vitamins, and its function is not entirely clear. It is necessary for growth and reproduction in animals and probably in human beings. From 25 to 30 units of vitamin E has recently been established as the recommended daily allowance. It is found naturally in green leaves and cereal seeds, especially wheat germ. It is also present in corn, soybean, and cottonseed oils. Small amounts are found in milk, butter, eggs, and liver. Diets that include whole-grain cereals and breads, milk, eggs, and leafy green vegetables are unlikely to be deficient in vitamin E.

The requirement for vitamin E appears to be increased if a large amount of unsaturated fat is included in the diet. Of course, many of the sources of unsaturated fat, such as vegetable oil, will also contain some vitamin E if stored properly. The recommended allowance stated here is adequate to cover a generous intake of unsaturated fat.

VITAMIN C

Although this vitamin is probably taken by more people as a supplement than other vitamins, it is found in many delicious natural foods—oranges, grapefruit, tomatoes, peppers, melons, and many other fruits and vegetables. It is destroyed by exposure to heat and air and dissolves readily in water and juices of all kinds. It is added to most canned fruit juices in liberal quantities. Certainly there is no excuse for an American to be deficient in vitamin C if only the sources are well known.

Vitamin C is involved in the synthesis of collagen, which gives structure to skin, cartilage, tendons, ligaments, blood vessels, bones, and teeth. It also enhances the absorption of iron. It is generally taken in much greater quantities than is probably necessary to maintain the adequate body pool of about 1500 milligrams. Any excess taken is lost in the urine.

The minimum amount required in the daily diet is about 35 milligrams, and the National Research Council has recommended a daily intake of at least 55 to 60 milligrams to allow a margin for error. This amount can be obtained from ½ cup of orange or grapefruit juice. It can be taken in a variety of other combinations of fruits and vegetables as well. Your diabetic diet will contain a specific number of fruits and vegetables. It is important to take these from the specified foods in order to ensure adequate vitamin C. Like the B vitamins, C comes with carbohydrate attached, and it is, therefore, important that the diabetic get as much vitamin as possible for the amount of carbohydrate. If your diet was planned by a dietitian or a physician, provision will have been made for adequate vitamin C.

B VITAMINS

This group encompasses a wide variety of compounds that are found in dissimilar places and perform a wide range of biologic duties. All are necessary in small amounts for good health, growth, and reproduction. Most come with considerable carbohydrate attached, and it is therefore necessary to make all carbohydrate foods as nutritious in B vitamins as possible. Many of these vitamins may be obtained from frequently eaten foods such as bread, but others are found in seldom eaten foods such as liver and wheat germ.

Enrichment of white flour adds vitamin B_1, riboflavin, niacin, and iron in amounts that approximate the content of those substances in whole-wheat flour. This provides a reasonable facsimile of whole-wheat flour for the person who prefers white bread and who may take unlimited amounts of bread and other foodstuffs daily. Such an option is not available to many diabetics, however. In addition to the above-mentioned nutrients, whole wheat contains folic acid, biotin, inositol, and para-aminobenzoic acid—all part of the B complex and necessary for good health. All these nutrients can be obtained from other sources, but if the carbohydrate intake is limited to 150 grams per day or less, it may not be possible to obtain the nutrients and remain within the recommended amount of carbohydrate. For this reason, and because mineral content is seriously impaired by the milling process used to make white flour, the Committee on Food and Nutrition of the American Diabetes Association has recommended that diabetics use whole-grain breads and cereals.

The increased fiber content of whole-grain cereals has a favorable effect on blood-sugar levels. It also aids elimination.

On the other hand, one must not entirely sacrifice enjoyment of food to the pursuit of good nutrition, nor is it necessary to do so. Certain dishes do not lend themselves well to the use of whole-wheat flour. In these few dishes, then, one should seek methods of supplementing white flour without altering the flavor. This can often be done by substituting other flours, such as soy, for a portion of the total flour. Another method is to sift ¼ cup brewer's yeast with 2 cups of white flour, an addition that increases the flour's nutritional level considerably and alters its flavor hardly at all. If such flour is then used for baking bread, crust, dumplings, or pastries, the flavor of the yeast is entirely compatible. Some nutritionists feel the above precautions are unnecessary, but I believe this kind of supplementation is better nutritionally (and financially) than the multiple-vitamin tablets so widely taken.

B vitamins are found in the seeds of most plants; for example, dried beans, peas, and nuts all contain differing amounts of the various compounds. Liver and brewer's yeast are excellent sources of B vitamins. However, for most people, bread and cereal will remain the primary sources of B vitamins, and we must be sure that the bread eaten is of the highest nutritional quality.

THIAMIN (B_1)

Thiamin (B_1) is involved in energy metabolism. It promotes the use of carbohydrate and contributes to normal functioning of the nerves. The requirement varies with the number of calories eaten. Adults will need about ½ milligram for each 1000 calories eaten. Pork is an excellent source. Lamb, liver, and legumes contain good amounts, while beef, chicken, fish, whole-grain cereals, leafy vegetables, and milk contain fair amounts.

RIBOFLAVIN

Riboflavin (B_2) is necessary for normal energy and protein metabolism in skin, eyes, and other body tissues. It is found in especially generous amounts in liver and milk. Eggs, dairy products, leafy vegetables, meat, fish, and poultry are also good sources.

NIACIN

Niacin is necessary for proper utilization of fat and carbohydrate. It is used in enzyme systems in the skin, nerves, and digestive tract. Liver, meat, fish, poultry, and nuts are excellent sources. Legumes and whole-grain cereals are also good sources. The recommended allowance is about 13 milligrams daily.

VITAMIN B_{12}

Vitamin B_{12} deficiency is ordinarily seen only in strict vegetarians, because it is present primarily in meat and meat products. It can, however, also occur in patients who have had stomach or bowel surgery and certain parasitic diseases. It occurs in these situations because the absorption is altered. When a deficiency exists, anemia will result, as will malfunction of the nerves to the feet and legs. Vitamin supplements will aid the vegetarian but will not affect those patients with difficulty in absorption, who will need to take the vitamin by injection. The recommended daily allowance is 3 micrograms for adults.

PYRIDOXINE (VITAMIN B₆)

Pyridoxine is necessary for normal energy and protein metabolism. Deficiencies have also been reported in women taking oral contraceptives. The best sources of this vitamin are liver, legumes, and whole-grain products. The recommended daily allowance is 2 milligrams daily for adults. If an oral contraceptive or other form of estrogen is taken for prolonged periods, a supplement may be needed.

FOLIC ACID

Folic acid is necessary for normal blood formation and normal nerve function. Good sources include liver, leafy vegetables, fruit, and brewer's yeast. It should be noted that deficiencies can sometimes be caused by oral contraceptives, so if anemia occurs when these compounds are taken, a supplement may be needed. The recommended daily allowance is 400 micrograms.

PANTOTHENIC ACID

Pantothenic acid is involved in energy and fat metabolism. It is present in liver, eggs, meat, fish, poultry, whole-grain products, and milk. No daily requirement has been determined. A daily intake of 10 milligrams is probably adequate.

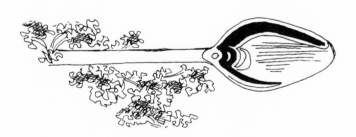

CHAPTER 3

Planning Ahead

- Biscuit Mix
- Egg Noodles
- Corn Bread Mix
- Pie Crust Mix
- Meat Loaves

- Quick Spaghetti Sauce
- Pancake Mix
- Bran Muffin Mix
- Lemonade Base
- Medego Villari

Diabetics, perhaps more than any other people, should pay attention to meal planning. Many people who find dieting a hassle might comply with their medical advice more readily if they understood how much a good meal plan can simplify life. "Meal planning" sounds like such work! It shouldn't be. I did it for years before I considered it in these formal terms, but there is no way that I or thousands of other women like me, and many men too, could cope with professional and home life simultaneously without this skill. Anyone can master it. First of all, PLAN AHEAD. Use the time increment that works for you, a week, a month, or whatever.

If Monday is always a hazard to your health, and a day more pressing than most, take 10 minutes on Sunday night to mix yourself a breakfast drink that can be poured in the blender and sipped while you dress. Make a sack lunch and leave it in the refrigerator overnight to eat at your desk or wherever you find yourself at lunch. Take a prepared casserole out of the freezer for your evening meal. When you get home, just put your casserole in the oven, set the timer, and put your feet up while it warms. But, you say, there is no casserole in the freezer (or God forbid, no freezer), and that of course is what planning ahead is all about.

Since we must start somewhere, let us start with an empty pantry on the day after payday. Take half an hour and plan seven breakfasts, lunches, and dinners. Consider which days you have time to cook leisurely meals and which days you are in a rush all day. Adjust the meals accordingly. The most common reason I hear for meal skipping or junk-food eating is "I'm just too tired to fix a meal after work." The feeling is familiar to most of us, but it's an indulgence that a diabetic cannot afford. Having made the menus, prepare a shopping list that will provide every necessary ingredient for meal preparation. If you have a big freezer, this can be done once a month instead of once a week.

When you are home from the grocery store, wash your salad greens, drain them well, and prepare a large bowl of tossed salad. Do not include the dressing or soft fruits and vegetables such as tomatoes. Those will be added at the last minute. Cover the entire bowl with plastic wrap and put it in the refrigerator. Each night you can remove a portion and dress it at serving time. A freshly tossed salad is ideal, but this is far better than no salad at all. Look at your menus and determine whether some of the things can be cooked ahead. Most casserole dishes warm up without too much loss in nutrition and taste. They will also keep easily for a week in the refrigerator, if they are kept covered and transferred there directly after cooking and cooling.

If you are having baked chicken, meat loaf, and tuna casserole all in one week, cook them all at once. You save cleaning time, cooking time, energy, and money. Then there will be a casserole to remove from the freezer when needed.

Microwave ovens can be a lifesaver for warming such dishes, but a regular oven will work almost as well—it just takes longer. Actually, it's a waste of time to make just one meat loaf or one casserole. Always do more than one; eat one and freeze one for later. You'll eat better and work at it less, and it will be cheaper.

My delightful friend Karl Ruppert is a physician and a bachelor. He is the least compulsive person I know, but he does a good job of feeding himself and the multitudes that drop in and out of his place. He once carried the "prepare more than one thing at a time" idea to an all-time high. We were invited to his house for dinner one night and arrived to find no one home, not an unusual situation. We let ourselves in, as is the custom there, and soon the phone rang to tell us he was delayed somewhere and please to be comfortable until he arrived. I started rummaging around the kitchen to see what he had in mind for dinner and came upon the entrée or I should say entrées. There in a giant roasting pan were three chickens, a pot roast, and a pork shoulder. The chicken was for dinner, and the others were simply being cooked for later!

I love cooking but hate cleaning up, so over the years I have tended to cook infrequently in great quantities; thus there is always something ready to eat and the kitchen gets really upset only once in a while.* One day, I had been on one of these cooking binges, having found a great bargain on frying chickens at the market. As the larder was empty of prepared-ahead meals, I began a cook-in of epic proportions. I made three meat loaves, and since they were going to be in the oven, I baked all seven of the fryers I had just bought. The ovens got the kitchen nice and warm, just right for raising bread, so three loaves of Savrud were started. By the time the Savrud was ready for the oven, the meat loaves and chicken were out. Maybe a casserole or two for the oven while the bread is baking?

A chicken, noodle, and green pea casserole! No noodles? No noodles! Let's see, one egg beaten well, a little salt, and enough flour to make a stiff dough. That done, the noodles were rolled and hung to dry over the rolling pin while the Chicken Divan casseroles were prepared.

Before the noodles were dry, and when about the kitchen sat 7 baked chickens, 3 meat loaves, 3 loaves of Savrud, fresh uncooked noodles, 2 casseroles, 1 bowl of poached chicken livers (salvaged from the fryers), 1 pot of stock, and a big bowl of dog food prepared from the giblets and necks—the door bell rang. It was our friend Bette Crosby, followed soon by my husband and his golfing buddy Carl Reder. Son Jeffrey arrived straightaway. The food began to disappear. First, warm bread with butter, then warm bread with thick slices of meat loaf, chicken tails were pinched off, then wings, and so on.

The noodles were finally cooked and into a casserole for dinner—not that anyone needed dinner at that point! A simple case of the best-laid plans going far astray!

Mixes

Our planning-ahead discussion would not be complete without some mention of prepared mixes. There are many very good mixes available

---

*My husband says this is a plain misstatement of fact! He says I can wreck the kitchen warming a casserole or boiling an egg. Alas, it's true!

on the market commercially, but it is also possible to make your own. For a diabetic this makes good nutritional sense. That way, you don't wonder how much carbohydrate or fat is present; you know. (The food processor is a great innovation for preparing these staples.) I'm including those things I have found useful as well as some contributed by mothers of larger families. These will keep fresher longer if stored in the freezer or refrigerator.

BISCUIT MIX

3 cups flour
1/3 cup butter, margarine, or other
   solid fat

2 tablespoons baking powder
1 1/2 teaspoons salt

Combine dry ingredients and mix well. Add fat and cut in well. Store in a plastic bag or airtight container in freezer or refrigerator.

To make biscuits from this mix, combine 1 cup of mix with 1/3 cup buttermilk. Bake in a very hot oven at 475° for 10 minutes or until well browned.

This mix can be substituted for prepared biscuit mix in any recipe.

Each cup of mix (12 biscuits) contains: 92 grams carbohydrate, 18 grams protein, and 13 grams fat.

Each biscuit contains: 8 grams carbohydrate, 1 gram protein, and 1 gram fat.

Exchange value: Each biscuit = 1 bread exchange.

EGG NOODLES

1 egg
1/2 cup flour

1/4 teaspoon salt

Mix well and roll out as thin as possible on a floured surface. When dough has been rolled into a large sheet, let it dry for a few minutes before cutting into desired shapes. It can be cut into 3-inch squares and used as won ton noodles or any meat- or cheese-filled noodle.

This is a high-protein and nutritious substitute for regular commercial noodles. Vegetarians are encouraged to use these noodles instead of the commercial variety. When the budget is slim and the meat is being stretched as far as possible, this noodle will supplement protein for good nutrition. These noodles can be frozen for future use or can be stored in a jar in your cupboard if they are thoroughly dried. Larger amounts can be prepared by doubling or tripling the ingredients. Serves 2.

Total recipe contains: 42 grams carbohydrate, 13 grams protein, 7 grams fat, and 273 calories.

Exchange value: 1 serving (½ total) = 1½ bread and 1 meat.

If you use commercially available noodles, I recommend soy noodles, or if these are not available, use egg noodles because of their relatively high content of protein and other nutrients.

CORN BREAD MIX

1 cup cornmeal
1 cup wheat germ
1 cup flour

2 tablespoons baking powder
1½ teaspoons salt
⅓ cup oil

Mix the dry ingredients thoroughly, then add the oil. Mix and store in an airtight container in the refrigerator or freezer.

To make corn bread from this mix: combine 1 egg with ½ cup buttermilk. Mix with 1 cup of mix. Bake at 450° for 15 minutes or until brown. Serves 8.

This can be substituted for cornmeal mix in any recipe.

Each cup of mix contains: 103 grams carbohydrate, 26 grams protein, and 36 grams fat.

Exchange value: Each piece = 1 bread.

PIE CRUST MIX

4 cups flour
2 teaspoons salt

1½ cups shortening

Mix the dry ingredients. Cut in shortening.

Store in dry state; or add ½ cup plus 2 tablespoons ice water.

Roll out into four 8-inch pie shells. Freeze pie shells unbaked in aluminum tins, covered with plastic wrap.

Each cup of mix or 1 shell will contain: 90 grams carbohydrate, 18 grams protein, and 36 grams fat.

Exchange value: ⅛ shell = 1 bread.

MEAT LOAVES

1 cup rolled oats, uncooked	3 cloves garlic, grated
3 pounds hamburger	1 large onion, finely chopped
2 pounds pork sausage, bulk	1 large carrot, grated
1 cup wheat germ	3 stalks celery, finely chopped
3 eggs	1 green pepper, finely chopped
1 large can evaporated skim milk	½ teaspoon powdered ginger
2 tablespoons salt	¼ cup fresh chopped parsley

Mix everything together until well blended and form into three or four meat loaves. Bake at 350° for about 1½ hours or until done in center.

These will freeze well if wrapped tightly in aluminum foil and stored in a plastic bag. Thaw in refrigerator overnight and warm in a 225° oven for about 45 minutes. They can be thawed in the oven at the same temperature, but it will take a bit longer.

Exchange value: 1 ounce cooked loaf = 1 meat exchange.

QUICK SPAGHETTI SAUCE

1 jar (32 ounces) commercial spaghetti sauce	1 bunch parsley
½ teaspoon oregano	½ pound ground beef or pork, browned (optional)
2 cloves garlic, grated	
1 large can mushroom stems and pieces with liquid	

Combine ingredients. Add browned ground meat, well seasoned, if meat sauce is desired. Simmer until spaghetti is done.

One of the prepared meat loaves can be divided lengthwise and submerged in this sauce and simmered gently for a few minutes. Serve with noodles or a green vegetable and salad for a quick and easy meal.

Exchange value: 1 cup sauce = 1 vegetable.

PANCAKE MIX

3 cups flour	1½ teaspoons salt
2 tablespoons baking powder	1 tablespoon sugar

Mix well and store in an airtight container in freezer or refrigerator. Can be used in any recipe calling for pancake mix.

(continued)

Pancakes from Mix: 1 cup mix
                   1 egg
                   2 tablespoons oil
                   ½ cup buttermilk

Cook as usual. Makes 6 large pancakes.

Waffles from Mix: 1 cup mix
                 1 egg
                 1 tablespoon oil
                 ⅔ cup buttermilk

Cook as usual. Makes 2 waffles.

LOW-CHOLESTEROL NOTE: Egg substitutes can be used in this recipe if desired.

Crêpes from Mix: 1 cup mix
                1 egg
                4 tablespoons oil
                ¾ cup buttermilk

Cook as usual. Makes 10 crêpes.
    One cup mix contains 95 grams carbohydrate.

BRAN MUFFIN MIX

1 cup bran flakes	1 cup buttermilk
1 cup wheat germ	⅓ cup oil
1 cup whole-wheat flour	2 eggs
1 tablespoon baking powder	¼ cup sugar
1¼ teaspoons salt	

Mix bran flakes, wheat germ, flour, baking powder, and salt. Add buttermilk, oil, eggs, and sugar. Stir just until mixed.
    The mix can be stored in the refrigerator for 10 to 14 days.
    Bake in an oiled muffin tin at 350° for 25 minutes. Makes 18 large muffins or 24 small ones. Each muffin will contain: 10 grams carbohy-

drate, 3 grams protein, and 5 grams fat.

Exchange value: 1 large muffin = 1 bread.

LEMONADE BASE

1½ cups lemon juice
1 fresh lemon, thinly sliced
½ cup boiling water

Sugar substitute equivalent to 1½
cups sugar

Put the sliced lemon and boiling water in a covered refrigerator jar. Press the slices with the back of a wooden spoon until they are bruised. Add the lemon juice and sweetener. Keep in the refrigerator until ready to use.

For 1 glass of lemonade, combine 4 tablespoons (¼ cup) mix in ½ glass water. Add ice cubes, stir, and serve with one of the slices from the bottom of the jar.

Total recipe contains: 39 grams carbohydrate, 3 grams protein, and 1 gram fat.

1 serving (⅛ total) contains: 5 grams carbohydrate.

Exchange value: One serving = ½ fruit.

MEDEGO VILLARI

2 cups bread crumbs
1 bunch parsley, very finely
chopped
1 medium onion, very finely
chopped

2 cloves garlic, grated
½ cup Parmesan or Romano
cheese

Mix all ingredients and store in an airtight container or plastic bag in the freezer. Use for bread crumbs or oven-fried foods. Chicken can be coated with a film of oil and rolled in these crumbs. It's delicious if baked at about 325° until brown. We have used this mix in the Baked Red Peppers (page 120), Spinach Pie (page 123), and several other dishes included elsewhere in this book.

Total recipe contains: 100 grams carbohydrate, 42 grams protein, 24 grams fat, and 784 calories.

(continued)

COMMENT: It's hard to let this recipe pass without commenting on its history. For years, I have salvaged old bread and bits of parsley, leftover onion, and so forth, and used them in a similar mix. It has always been a "floating mix" that was never the same twice. I just continuously added to it as I had an extra ingredient left over from some other meal preparation. My husband has commented that it was hard to reconcile apparent contradictions in the character of a lady who could buy a fur coat on one hand and save little pieces of onion on the other. I have always replied that I would much rather have a new coat than a new onion. My mix never had a name.

To my surprise, once while visiting in the home of Evelyn and Dominic (Val) Villari, Val was busy preparing a similar mix from perfectly new and good ingredients. No leftover business here. He was using a whole new bunch of parsley, a new onion, etc. "What are you making?" said I. "Medego," said Villari. So, when cookbook revision time came, I wanted to include this mixture, and since his was a more precise mixture, and had a name, his recipe was requested.

First, I asked, "How do you spell medego?" "Gosh, I never saw it spelled," he said. He would call his sister in Rhode Island, he promised. She would know. My second telephone call to California requesting the spelling was met with gales of laughter from Evelyn. There is no such word, I was told. When little Dominic Villari used to see his mother dip slices of veal or fish in beaten egg and dredge them in this bread crumb mix and would ask, like little boys the world over, "What is that stuff, Mom?," she would reply in the Italian idiom, "Soggy bread!" Now I suppose I will receive a dozen letters telling me that there is such a word and how to spell it, but that will have to wait for the Third Edition. For now, we will make do with my phonetic rendition of Mrs. Villari's Italian word meaning "soggy bread."

Meal Planning

In my experience the only system of meal planning that works is one that incorporates both my work schedule and a shopping list. A good meal-planning system should save more time than it takes to make the plan. In addition, it should take into account the time available to prepare the meal, the amount of money required to buy the ingredients, special individual needs (such as diabetics have), and, of course, nutritional content.

A serviceable plan might be as follows:

Step 1. Prepare a master list of main dishes, vegetables, breads, salads, and desserts served repeatedly to your family. It is desirable to subdivide the vegetable list into exchange or percentage lists.

Step 2. Combine the above components into meal plans, considering compatibility of preparation, flavor combinations, and the limitations of your diet.

Step 3. Make daily meal plans, considering three main meals and snacks, if any. If there are days when you arrive home late and wish to fix quick suppers, or mornings when you leave early and need quick breakfasts, be sure to consider these factors when making your daily plans. If your schedule is unpredictable, prepare a reserve of quick menus that can be easily altered to complete the day's nutritional needs.

Step 4. Check food content lists to be sure all essential nutrients are supplied each day and adjust as necessary. Clear soups, "3 percent" vegetables, and salads are useful to complete vitamin and mineral requirements when the day's allotments of carbohydrate, protein, fat, and calories have been used.

Step 5. Calculate the carbohydrate, protein, and fat content of each individual dish if you are dealing with a weighed diet, or of exchanges in the case of an exchange diet. If a permanent record is made of these calculations, they need to be computed only once. Add each day's total of these components and adjust to fit the diet prescription. It will be necessary to rearrange meal plans, substituting a lower-carbohydrate vegetable or adding extra protein to the main dish, in some cases. Check the distribution of food throughout the day and be certain that not more than one-third of the total daily allowance is taken at any one meal.

Step 6. Next to the meal plans, list each ingredient needed to prepare each dish. Take a separate sheet of paper and list those ingredients that you do not now have on hand. This becomes your grocery shopping list. Consider the example in Table 4. If this method is followed, frequent trips to the grocery store are unnecessary, and considerable money is saved as the result. In addition, you always have what is needed to prepare each meal.

In practice, only Step 6 need be done more than once. Thus, considerable time is saved, not only shopping time but planning time as well. The diet prescription can be easily worked into the family meal plan, and you can be assured that nutritional needs are being met.

TABLE 4. SAMPLE DAILY MEAL PLAN

Diet prescription
    8 meat exchanges
    3 fruit exchanges
    3 milk exchanges
    3 group A vegetable exchanges
    2 bread exchanges
    4 fat exchanges

Menus	Chores	Shopping List
	Breakfast	
Scrambled eggs	Thaw ground meat for	1 dozen eggs
Bran muffins	dinner	1 box bran flakes
Milk		1 quart fresh milk
Strawberries and "cream"		Strawberries
		Evaporated skim milk
	Lunch	
Crab salad	Make gelatin dessert,	Crab
Spinach soup	using strawberries	Spinach
Milk	from breakfast	Cantaloupe
Cantaloupe		
	Dinner	
Meat loaf		Ground meat
Green beans		Green beans
Cole slaw		Cabbage
Corn bread		Cornmeal
Strawberry gelatin dessert		Sugar-free gelatin
Milk		

SPECIAL PROBLEMS

Some special problems must be taken into account when dealing with diabetic diets. Some of these are considered here, and others are discussed in Chapter 10.

DELAYED MEALS

Diabetics who take insulin, and to a lesser degree those who take the oral medications, must maintain a reasonably regular meal schedule. If this is altered to a significant degree, hypoglycemia results. Unfortunately, the evening meal is the one most often delayed, and this is also the time of day when hypoglycemia is most likely to occur.

The danger is avoided most simply if the meal plan includes a nutritious beverage such as milk. Then, if the meal cooks slower than anticipated or if there is some interruption, the beverage can be taken by the diabetic member without disruption of the meal plan, and an insulin reaction can be averted. One should never wait, hoping that dinner will be ready before hypoglycemia occurs. Rather, hypoglycemia should be expected and avoided, since it is not only unpleasant but often harmful.

UNEXPECTED VISITORS

Not infrequently, people drop by unexpectedly and do not wish to stay for a meal. The diabetic may be embarrassed to interrupt the visit. Again, the problem can be avoided by including in each meal plan a glass of milk or other nutritious beverage that can be quickly taken by the diabetic member, avoiding both discomfort and physiologic unrest.

EATING IN RESTAURANTS

The most difficult thing to avoid in restaurant meals is extra fat. It is camouflaged in many ways, and you can consume considerable quantities without realizing it. Remember that shellfish, fish, and fowl contain the least amounts of inherent fat. Therefore, if extra fat is added in cooking, the total will be less than if you begin with a high-fat meat, such as beef or pork, and then add more. So, order seafood, preferably steamed, broiled, or poached. Request that salad dressings be served separately, so you can more carefully gauge the total amount than if it is already on the salad.

Carbohydrate is also generously served but is more easily recognized because of its bulk. If your carbohydrate allowance does not permit both bread and potato, request a substitute vegetable if potato is served. Most restaurants have beets and green beans available. Virtually all restaurants have a food scale available, and portions can be weighed if requested, but if you know your diet well, this should not be necessary.

COCKTAIL PARTIES

These pose a triple threat—alcohol, snacks, and impaired judgment. Physicians are by no means in complete accord about permitting alcohol for diabetics. Those who permit it generally allow only hard liquor, such as whiskey, in very limited amounts, and forbid beer and wine. American beer usually contains about 4 percent carbohydrate, which must be counted in the dietary calculations. Wine may contain a considerable amount of unfermented sugar and must not be taken. Whiskeys do not contain carbohydrate and are therefore often permitted.

It is well to remember that the body cannot metabolize more than about 10 milliliters of alcohol per hour (that is about the quantity in an ounce of whiskey), and it is therefore not wise to drink more than that amount. The alcohol in whiskey represents about 70 calories per ounce, and these calories must be counted, especially if weight control is a problem. A noncaloric mixer, such as plain water, soda, or diet quinine water, may be used freely. Many mixes contain sugar, so read the label.

Impaired judgment can be avoided if the rule of 1 ounce of whiskey an hour is adhered to strictly. A good way to do this is to order a tall, diluted drink and sip it slowly. This does not induce the alcoholic euphoria so widely desired, but it does prevent hangovers.

Snacks can be taken in moderation, provided judgment is not impaired. Unfortunately, ordinarily reasonable alternatives in the forms of celery sticks, tomatoes, and carrot strips are completely offset by the high-fat mixtures they are either stuffed with or dipped into. It takes an extraordinary amount of self-control to eat a plain carrot strip when there is a bowl of cheese dip within reach. If it is your cocktail party, don't make the dip. If it is your friend's party, do your best with self-control. On the other hand, when the meal is delayed, snacks may actually be the means to avoid hypoglycemia, and if you suspect the meal may not be served on time, snack judiciously. Avoid snacks obviously high in carbohydrate and fat. These include dips of all kinds, cheese, sausages, and olives. Some pickles are quite sweet and must be avoided. Stick to the vegetables, if any; if none, small crackers in reasonable number can usually be compensated for at the evening meal (see Table 5 for exchange values of snack crackers).

TABLE 5. CRACKER EXCHANGE VALUES

Type	Amount	Exchange value
Bacon thins	15	1 bread, 2 fat
Blue cheese	12	1 bread, 1 fat
Cheese tidbits	30	½ bread
Chippers, potato or bacon	8	1 bread, 1 fat
French onion thins	12	1 bread, 1 fat
Ritz	7	1 bread, 1 fat
Rye Thins	10	1 bread, 1 fat
Ry-Krisp	3	1 bread
Sesame Thins	10	1 bread, 2 fat
Toasted three-ring pretzels	6	1 bread
Triangle Thins	15	1 bread, 1 fat
Triscuits	5	1 bread, 1 fat
Veri-Thin pretzel sticks	30	½ bread
Wheat thins	12	1 bread

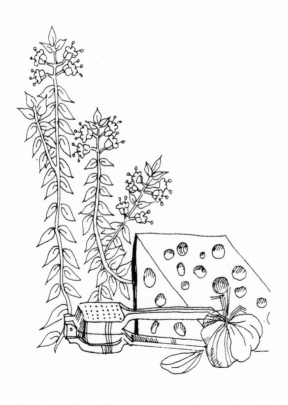

CHAPTER 4

Food Preparation

There will be no attempt to teach basic cooking techniques in this book, since diabetics may prepare their food by all available methods. However, there are certain techniques that tend to conserve nutrients and others that needlessly destroy them, and these will be described. Vitamins and minerals are important because many diabetics must limit their caloric intake, and every effort should be made to conserve as many nutrients as possible.

Juices that escape during the preparation of meats and vegetables contain many vitamins and minerals and should be retained and used in some manner. Meat juices can be utilized in sauces, dips, and soups. They often contain B vitamins, as well as iron, potassium, and other minerals. Ingenious cooks will have no problem disposing of these juices in a flavorful manner.

Many recipes call for soaking vegetables and suggest that the soaking water be discarded. If you have such a recipe in your files, discard it instead of the soaking water. All vegetables should have only a passing acquaintance with water prior to cooking. Except for leafy vegetables, which may contain sand, most vegetables can be rinsed rapidly with cold water and cooked immediately. All B vitamins dissolve easily in water and can consequently be lost forever if either the soaking or the cooking water is discarded. The cooking water (or pot liquor) can be used as a soup or broth or added to other juices with compatible flavors. If you do not use the cooking water in this way, use it as a cooking liquid for other dishes; don't discard it. Such cooking liquid is especially important if you must take additional potassium in your diet. Most of the potassium present in food is lost in cooking water.

COOKING METHODS

There are several methods of cooking vegetables that are unfamiliar to many Americans but have much to recommend them with regard to both flavor and nutrition.

Butter-steaming requires the use of a heavy pot with a tight-fitting lid and a rack to hold the vegetables aloft. Add as generous an amount of butter or margarine as your diet will allow and place the vegetables on the rack. Add ¼ cup of water in the bottom of the pan and cook on medium heat. Since there is almost no liquid, few nutrients are lost. The water should not be permitted to touch the vegetables.

Stir-frying, a method used by Oriental cooks, utilizes a wok, a heavy frying pan, or an electric skillet and a very small amount of cooking oil. The oil is heated quite hot, and the sliced vegetables are rapidly stirred while they are seared by the hot pan. The high heat caramelizes some of the starch in the vegetables and results in a surprisingly good flavor.

Waterless cooking can be accomplished with any heavy pan and a tight-fitting lid. This method uses the water already present in the vegetables by preventing its evaporation: they steam in their own juice. A somewhat lower cooking temperature is necessary to avoid scorching the food.

Regardless of the method used, the quicker the cooking can be accomplished, the fewer nutrients are lost. Likewise, smaller amounts of liquid are preferable to larger amounts, unless leftover liquid can be used to advantage.

Low-fat diets sometimes require special cooking techniques. The specially coated pans are good for sautéing with little or no fat. These are marketed under a number of trade names.

Microwave ovens have revolutionized cooking in many American kitchens. We have not included microwave techniques in our recipes, but most could be adapted to that technique. This method has much to recommend it in time and energy savings, and it adapts especially well to low-fat cookery.

Food processors are the current rage in kitchens that can afford them. You will find several recipes that recommend the use of this appliance. In most of them a blender or mixer could be used with equally good results. We have simply recommended the particular appliance that we used to test the recipe. I confess to having been very skeptical of the advertising claims made for the food processor, but I found it invaluable while testing and retesting the many recipes necessary for this book, and now I am an enthusiastic convert.

SEASONINGS

Any kind of seasoning can be used by diabetic patients. The only possible restriction is frequent use of wine and liquors. Both are used much more commonly in American kitchens than when the first edition of this book was written. If a wine sauce is simmered, it will not be necessary to include the alcohol in your calculations; it will evaporate. But the carbohydrate will remain and must be included. When dishes are flamed—for example, with brandy—the brandy can be ignored, as again the alcohol will be burned off. Usually it will be necessary to include a little sugar to flame properly, and this too can be ignored.

TABLE 6. CARBOHYDRATE CONTENT OF 1 OUNCE OF WINE

Wine	Carbohydrate (grams)	Alcohol (grams)	Calories
Brandy	0	10.5	73
Port	3.5	4.0	40
Sauterne	1.0	2.5	22
Sherry	2.4	4.5	30

SUGAR SUBSTITUTES

Although sugar must be avoided by diabetics, a number of other sweetening agents are available. These vary widely in sweetening ability and composition. It is best to rely on the manufacturer's instructions when substituting in a recipe. Although these products are marketed under a variety of trade names, they contain one of the compounds listed below. Consult the label on your favorite product to see what the sweetening agent is.

Saccharin is the oldest of the noncaloric sweeteners. It has many times the sweetening power of sugar and must be used in small amounts. For many people, saccharin has an unpleasant, bitter aftertaste, and when these people are also diabetic, it is unfortunate indeed. Saccharin is available in tablet and liquid form and can be used as directed on the package. It is not suitable for foods that must be cooked or frozen after the sweetener is added, as definite alteration of taste and loss of sweetness occurs. It is most satisfactory when added immediately before serving. Saccharin is not available in Canada.

Cyclamates offered a pleasant alternative to those who found saccharin unpalatable. Although there was no evidence that these compounds were harmful to human beings in amounts customarily used by diabetic patients, they have been ordered off the market by the Food and Drug Administration. This decision was based on animal experiments that suggested that large doses might be harmful. Consequently, no recipes using this substance are included here. Cyclamate can still be purchased in Canada.

Sorbitol is commonly found in the "dietetic" candies and gums. It is a carbohydrate and must be counted, both as carbohydrate and calories (4 calories per gram), in the diabetic diet. It causes little change in the blood-sugar level and may be used in moderation by diabetics.

Lactose has only moderate sweetening ability and is sometimes combined with saccharin in commercial "artificial sugars." Like sorbitol, it can be used by diabetics, provided it is calculated as carbohydrate in the diet. These artificial sugars replace sugar on a volume-for-volume basis. This has obvious advantages to the cook who is trying to adapt a recipe, although such substitutions are not always successful. The artificial sugars have the disadvantage of being outrageously expensive and should be kept for special recipes. They are especially good for garnishing fresh fruits, because they give the appearance of powdered sugar. About half of the lactose forms ordinary sugar as it is broken down in digestion, and some physicians object to it for this reason. Ask your physician for an opinion if you want to use significant amounts of these sweeteners.

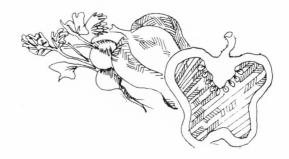

CHAPTER 5

Appetizers

- **Ted Branscome's Artichokes**
- **Mushrooms Medego**
- **Stuffed Mushrooms**
- **Celery and Mushroom Sticks**
- **Cheese with Chutney**
- **Marinated Cheese**
- **Salmon and Cucumber Canapés**

- **Evelyn's Chicken Liver Pâté**
- **Desperation Liver Pâté**
- **Shrimp in Tomatoes**
- **Crab Ball**
- **Oyster Canapés**
- **Barbecued Pork**

TED BRANSCOME'S ARTICHOKES

1 large artichoke
2 tablespoons prepared French
  dressing, warmed

1 tablespoon melted butter

Steam artichoke, drain, and remove choke. Trim the bottom so it will sit comfortably in a shallow serving dish.

Combine the French dressing and melted butter and pour into the center well left by removing the choke. Drizzle a little into the openings between leaves. Leaves can be removed and eaten individually. Each will carry a bit of the "dip." Very good. Provide a small basket alongside for the discarded leaves. Serves 4 as an appetizer.

Total recipe contains: 15 grams carbohydrate, 3 grams protein, 22 grams fat, and 258 calories.

One serving (¼ of total) contains: 4 grams carbohydrate, 1 gram protein, 6 grams fat, and 64 calories.

Exchange value: 1 serving = ½ vegetable and 1 fat.

MUSHROOMS MEDEGO

2 dozen bite-size mushrooms
1 tablespoon oil
½ cup fine bread crumbs
1 boiled egg, very finely ground
1 tablespoon finely chopped onion

¼ teaspoon sage
¼ teaspoon ground black pepper
¼ cup chicken broth or drippings
   from a baked chicken

Remove stems from mushrooms and chop the stems finely. Combine the crumbs, egg, onion, and seasonings and mix thoroughly. Add chopped mushrooms. Add the broth, a tablespoon at a time, until the stuffing is just moist. You may not need all the broth, depending on your bread crumbs.

Toss the mushrooms with the oil until they are completely coated. Drain briefly on a paper towel. Fill the mushroom cavities with the stuffing mixture. Place on baking sheet. Bake at 400° for 10 minutes. Serve warm as appetizers. Serves 6.

Total recipe contains: 45 grams carbohydrate, 20 grams protein, 23 grams fat, and 461 calories.

One serving (⅙ of total) contains: 7 grams carbohydrate, 3 grams protein, 4 grams fat, and 77 calories.

Exchange value: 1 serving = about ½ bread and 1 fat.

STUFFED MUSHROOMS

8 mushrooms (2 to 3 inches in
   diameter)
1 teaspoon margarine, melted
2 green onions, chopped
2 medium tomatoes, peeled and
   chopped

½ teaspoon salt
2 tablespoons bread crumbs
¼ cup boiling water

Remove stems from mushrooms and chop the stems finely. Oil entire surface of mushrooms with melted margarine. Mix other ingredients, including chopped mushroom stems, and mound into mushroom caps. Place in flat pan and pour ¼ cup boiling water around caps. Bake in moderate oven (350°) for about 15 minutes. Serves 8.

Total recipe contains: 27 grams carbohydrate, 9 grams protein, and 4 grams fat.

Each mushroom contains: 3 grams carbohydrate, 1 gram protein, .5 gram fat, and 20 calories.

Exchange value: 1 mushroom = 1 Group A vegetable.

CELERY AND MUSHROOM STICKS

½ cup finely chopped raw   12 celery sticks
   mushrooms   3 tablespoons Low-Fat
¼ cup minced green pepper   Mayonnaise (page 67)

Blend mushrooms and green pepper with low-calorie mayonnaise and
fill celery sticks. Serve on lettuce or as hors d'oeuvres.
    Contains negligible carbohydrate, protein, and fat.

CHEESE WITH CHUTNEY

1 package (8 ounces) Neufchâtel   ¼ cup chutney
   cheese   1 green onion, finely chopped, or
½ teaspoon curry powder   chopped chives
1 tablespoon good dry sherry

Mix the cheese, curry, and sherry. Line bottom of a small rectangular
dish with plastic wrap and fill with the cheese mixture. Refrigerate until
quite firm. Lift cheese mixture from mold. Turn the cheese mixture
onto the serving plate and gently remove the plastic wrap. Spread the
chutney over the top and garnish with green onion or chopped chives.
Serve segments of celery, cucumber, or crisp crackers to accompany it.
Will serve about 8 as an appetizer.
    Total recipe contains: 42 grams carbohydrate, 17 grams protein, 48
grams fat, 2 grams alcohol, and 715 calories.
    One serving (⅛ of total) contains: 5 grams carbohydrate, 2 grams
protein, 6 grams fat, and 89 calories.
    Exchange value: 1 serving = about ½ fruit and 1 fat.

NOTE: If you have the patience, the appearance of this dish is much
improved by layering it as you might a torte—cheese, chutney, chives,
cheese, chutney, chives. In all modesty, it is an unattractive dish as
outlined above; good, but ugly!

MARINATED CHEESE

1 package (8 ounces) Neufchâtel
  cheese
¼ cup soy sauce
1 small clove garlic, grated

2 tablespoons toasted sesame
  seeds
A few chives

Open top of cheese wrapper and add the mixed soy sauce and garlic. Let rest in refrigerator until ready to serve.

Decant the sauce into a cup and place cheese in a shallow serving bowl. Surround with the liquid and top cheese with toasted sesame seeds and a few chives. Serve with crackers. Serves 16.

Total recipe contains: 18 grams carbohydrate, 21 grams protein, 62 grams fat, and 737 calories.

One serving (¹⁄₁₆ of total) contains: 1 gram carbohydrate, 1 gram protein, 4 grams fat, and 46 calories.

Exchange value: 1 serving = about 1 fat.

CALORIE-WISE NOTE: Use ricotta instead of Neufchâtel and save 500 calories.

SALMON AND CUCUMBER CANAPÉS

1 large English (or seedless)
  cucumber, sliced crosswise
1 can (7½ ounces) salmon
¼ cup finely chopped nuts

2 tablespoons Mayonnaise (page
  68)
Chopped parsley or parsley leaves
  for garnish

Combine the salmon, nuts, and mayonnaise and mix well. Top each cucumber slice with about 1 teaspoon of mixture and garnish with a little chopped parsley or a single leaf of parsley. Makes a pretty platter. Serves 12.

Total recipe contains: 11 grams carbohydrate, 57 grams protein, 65 grams fat, and 849 calories.

One serving (¹⁄₁₂ of total) contains: 1 gram carbohydrate, 8 grams protein, 5 grams fat, and 71 calories.

Exchange value: 1 serving = 1 medium-fat meat.

EVELYN'S CHICKEN LIVER PÂTÉ

1 pound chicken livers
1 onion
1 cup water
¾ cup diet margarine
4 tablespoons grated onion
2 teaspoons salt
¼ teaspoon pepper

¼ teaspoon mace
1½ teaspoons dry mustard
1 tablespoon brandy
3 hard-boiled eggs
Black pepper, chopped chives, or
    chopped parsley for garnish

Cook livers and onion in water until done. Remove livers, discard onion, and save the broth for the dog's dinner. Combine the liver and all the remaining ingredients in the food processor and work with the steel blade until it is smooth and creamy. Chill 3 to 4 hours.

Unmold and garnish with black pepper, chopped chives, or chopped parsley. Serve crackers, celery sticks, or sliced cucumbers alongside. Makes 2½ cups. Serves 20.

Total recipe contains: 17 grams carbohydrate, 121 grams protein, 109 grams fat, and 1524 calories.

One serving (¹⁄₂₀ of total) contains: 1 gram carbohydrate, 6 grams protein, 5 grams fat, and 76 calories.

Exchange value: 1 serving = about 1 medium-fat meat.

DESPERATION LIVER PÂTÉ

1 package (8 ounces) low-fat
    cream cheese
8 ounces of the best
    Braunschweiger available

2 green onions, finely chopped
2 teaspoons Worcestershire sauce
Chopped parsley or chives for
    garnish

Combine all ingredients except parsley in your mixer or food processor and mix thoroughly. Form into a mound on a serving dish. Garnish with parsley or chives. Serves 12.

Total recipe contains: 18 grams carbohydrate, 54 grams protein, 97 grams fat, and 1180 calories.

One serving (¹⁄₁₂ of total) contains: 1 gram carbohydrate, 5 grams protein, 8 grams fat, and 98 calories.

Exchange value: 1 serving = about 1 high-fat meat.

COMMENT: I call this Desperation Pâté because we do a lot of drop-in entertaining at our house and I have used this recipe so often it deserves a Medal of Honor. I usually serve it with celery segments.

SHRIMP IN TOMATOES

1 pound cherry tomatoes
2 cans (4½ ounces each) broken
  shrimp

1 green onion, chopped
1 tablespoon soy sauce
3 black olives, chopped

Slice off stem ends of tomatoes and scoop out pulp. Reserve for another use. Chop shrimp into tiny pieces and combine with soy sauce, onion, and olives. This can be done quickly in a blender or food processor. Fill tomato cavities. Serve as appetizers or on lettuce leaves as a salad. Serves 6.

Total recipe contains: 27 grams of carbohydrate, 60 grams of protein, 8 grams of fat, and 440 calories.

One serving (⅙ of total) contains: 5 grams carbohydrate, 10 grams protein, 1 gram fat, and 73 calories.

Exchange value: 1 serving = about 1 lean meat.

CRAB BALL

8 ounces Neufchâtel cheese
6¾ ounces Dungeness crab meat
  (canned or fresh)

1 tablespoon grated fresh onion
1 tablespoon chopped parsley

Combine ingredients and form into a ball. Refrigerate. Before serving, pour seafood cocktail sauce over crab ball. A nice appetizer when served with your favorite crackers. I especially like it with Ry-Krisp, Wheat Thins, and Triscuits. Best to let the ball set in the refrigerator at least several hours before serving. It seems to enhance the flavor. Serves 10.

Total recipe contains: 10 grams carbohydrate, 50 grams protein, 52 grams fat, and 740 calories.

One serving (⅒ of total) contains: 1 gram carbohydrate, 5 grams protein, 5 grams fat, and 74 calories.

Exchange value: 1 serving = 1 meat.

OYSTER CANAPÉS

1 pint fresh oysters   Salt and pepper
6 slices bacon, thinly sliced

Bring a pot of water to a rolling boil. Add a little salt and immerse the oysters, one at a time, for about one minute, remove, and drain. Cut oysters in quarters or halves, depending on size, and wrap each piece with a segment of bacon slice. Secure with a toothpick or a small skewer. Put on a rimmed baking sheet and bake at 350° for 8 to 10 minutes. Serves 8.

Total recipe contains: 29 grams carbohydrate, 53 grams protein, 23 grams fat, and 560 calories.

One serving (⅛ of total) contains: 4 grams carbohydrate, 7 grams protein, 3 grams fat, and 70 calories.

Exchange value: ½ medium-fat meat.

NOTE: Bette Crosby taught me this trick of poaching oysters before using in recipes. A flat oyster will quickly puff up and be firm enough to slice evenly.

BARBECUED PORK
(from the kitchen of Mrs. Thomas Chinn)

¼ cup soy sauce   ⅛ teaspoon ground cloves
2 tablespoons salad oil   1 pound lean pork roast (fat
⅛ teaspoon cayenne   trimmed off) or 3 pounds lean
⅛ teaspoon ground cinnamon   ribs

Cut pork into bite-size pieces. Combine ingredients in a plastic bag and marinate 1 to 2 hours. Remove meat from bag and discard marinade. Put meat on small rack or skewers and bake at 325° for 1 hour. Serve with hot mustard and toasted sesame seeds alongside for dipping. Serves 4.

Each ounce, about 6 pieces, of cooked pork contains: 7 grams protein, 5 grams fat, and 75 calories.

Exchange value: 1 serving = about 1 meat.

NOTE: When a marinade is discarded, it need not be counted in the calculations of food content.

CHAPTER 6

Salads and Salad Dressings

- **Crab Salad**
- **Tuna or Salmon Salad**
- **Asparagus Salad**
- **Cole Slaw**
- **Cucumber Marinade**
- **Marinated Mushrooms**
- **Stuffed Tomatoes**
- **Chinese Tomato Salad**

- **Molded Vegetable Salad**
- **Hawaiian Salad**
- **Low-Fat Mayonnaise**
- **Cheese Dressing**
- **Thousand Island Dressing**
- **Mayonnaise**
- **Fresh Herb Mayonnaise**
- **French Dressing**

CRAB SALAD

2 large tomatoes
1 teaspoon Mayonnaise (page 68)
1 tablespoon lemon juice
Several drops Tabasco
½ pound cooked crab meat
⅓ cup finely chopped celery

1 tablespoon finely chopped green onion
2 tablespoons chopped green pepper
½ teaspoon salt

Slice tomatoes and arrange on four salad plates (or two plates if this is the main course). Mix mayonnaise, lemon juice, and Tabasco together. Combine other ingredients. Add sauce and toss well. Place on top of tomato slices.

Entire recipe contains: 19 grams carbohydrate, 41 grams protein, and 10 grams fat. One-fourth of total (2¼ ounces) contains: 5 grams

61

carbohydrate, 10 grams protein, 2 grams fat, 80 calories
Exchange value: ¼ total = 1 Group A vegetable and 1½ meat.

TUNA OR SALMON SALAD

½ cup shredded cabbage
1 cup shredded tuna or cold
  cooked salmon
1 cup chopped walnuts
4 hard-cooked eggs, chopped

½ cup chopped sweet pickle
½ cup chopped celery
¼ cup Mayonnaise (page 68)
Salt and pepper to taste

Mix all ingredients except mayonnaise, salt, and pepper. Moisten with mayonnaise. Season to taste. Serves 6 as a salad or 4 as a main dish.

Entire recipe contains: 63.5 grams carbohydrate, 94 grams protein, 160 grams fat, and 2023 calories.

Exchange value: ¼ total = 1 bread, 3 medium-fat meat, and 5 fat; ⅙ total = ½ bread, 2 medium-fat meat, and 3 fat.

COMMENT: This is a super recipe for the dump-and-stir method of cooking. You can add lots more or lots less of almost any ingredient and it still tastes good, so when that extra person drops in at dinnertime, just put in more cabbage and celery and you have a bigger dinner salad. If you increase the fish, nuts, eggs, or mayonnaise, don't forget to increase the calculations proportionately. It goes well as a main dish with fresh hot Bran Muffins (page 42). If you must limit fat intake, Low-Fat Mayonnaise (page 67) can be used. In that case subtract 48 grams fat and 382 calories from total.

ASPARAGUS SALAD

4 cups fresh, raw asparagus tips
1 tablespoon Roquefort cheese
¼ cup vinegar

Salt and pepper
4 to 6 cups lettuce leaves

Slice asparagus tips diagonally. Crumble cheese into vinegar. Add salt and pepper to taste. Mix with asparagus. Serve on lettuce leaves. Yields 6 servings.

Total recipe contains: 28 grams carbohydrate, 17 grams protein, and 4 grams fat.

One cup serving contains: 5 grams carbohydrate, 3 grams protein, 1 gram fat, 40 calories, and generous amounts vitamin A.

Exchange value: 1 serving = about 1 Group A vegetable.

COLE SLAW

1 tablespoon finely chopped onion	¼ teaspoon salt
2 teaspoons prepared mustard	2 cups finely shredded cabbage
1 tablespoon Low-Fat Mayonnaise (page 67)	Toasted sesame seeds or toasted wheat germ for garnish

Mix dressing ingredients and toss with cabbage. Garnish with sesame seeds or wheat germ. Serves 4.

Total recipe contains: 11 grams carbohydrate, 4 grams protein, 0 grams fat.

1 serving (½ cup) contains: 3 grams carbohydrate, and vitamin C.

Exchange value: 1 Group A vegetable.

CUCUMBER MARINADE

1 large cucumber, sliced crosswise	Pinch of paprika
1 small green onion with top	2 drops liquid sweetener
½ teaspoon salt	1 tablespoon vinegar
Pinch of black pepper	¼ cup buttermilk

Combine all ingredients and chill for 15 minutes. Drain before serving. It need not be counted in daily diet calculations.

MARINATED MUSHROOMS

½ pound fresh mushrooms	1 small green onion, sliced
⅓ cup shallot red wine vinegar	1 tomato
1 teaspoon granular chicken bouillon	1 tablespoon chopped parsley
1 teaspoon dried savory	¼ cup water
	Crisp lettuce leaves

Mix and simmer all ingredients except lettuce for 5 minutes. Drain and serve on crisp lettuce leaves. Serves 4.

(continued)

Total recipe contains: 19 grams carbohydrate, 7 grams protein, and 0 grams fat.

One serving (¼ cup) contains: 5 grams carbohydrate, 2 grams protein, 25 calories, and vitamins A, B, C.

Exchange value: 1 serving = 1 Group A vegetable.

COMMENT: When instructions are given to drain away the liquid, as in the above recipe, it goes without saying that this liquid should be retained and used in some manner. Add to other marinades or soups, but do not discard.

STUFFED TOMATOES

4 large tomatoes
1 bunch water cress
1 small cucumber, diced

1 green onion, finely chopped
½ teaspoon salt
¼ teaspoon black pepper

Remove tomato pulp and mix with other ingredients. Stuff tomatoes. Makes four servings.

Total recipe contains: 10 grams carbohydrate, 2 grams protein, 50 calories per tomato, and vitamins A, B, C.

Exchange value: 1 Group B vegetable.

CHINESE TOMATO SALAD

½ teaspoon dry mustard
1 tablespoon soy sauce
1 teaspoon sesame oil
½ teaspoon salt

1 teaspoon water
2 cups cabbage, finely chopped
2 medium tomatoes, finely
  chopped

Blend mustard, soy sauce, sesame oil, salt, and water until smooth. Mix cabbage and tomatoes. Drizzle dressing over this. Serves 6.

Total recipe contains: 23 grams carbohydrate, 6 grams protein, and 5 grams fat.

One serving (½ cup) contains: 4 grams carbohydrate, 0 grams protein, 1 gram fat, 25 calories, and vitamins A, B, C.

Exchange value: 1 serving = 1 Group A vegetable.

MOLDED VEGETABLE SALAD

1 package sugar-free lemon
  gelatin dessert mix
2 cups boiling water
2 tablespoons fresh lemon juice

⅔ cup cabbage, chopped
⅔ cup green pepper, chopped
2 slices pimiento
Lettuce leaves

Dissolve gelatin dessert mix in boiling water and stir until completely dissolved. Add lemon juice. Add chopped vegetables and chill. Slice when firm and serve on lettuce leaves with low-calorie dressing.

Total recipe contains: 8 grams carbohydrate, 7 grams protein, and 0 grams fat.

One serving contains: negligible amounts carbohydrate, protein, and fat; 20 calories; and large amounts vitamins A and C.

It need not be included in diet calculations.

HAWAIIAN SALAD

¼ teaspoon salt
1 cup thinly sliced cucumbers
½ cup thinly sliced carrots
½ cup thinly sliced mushrooms
  (optional)

⅛ teaspoon ground ginger
¼ cup white wine vinegar
2 drops liquid sweetener

Add salt to cucumbers and let stand for 10 minutes. Add remainder of ingredients. Chill in refrigerator for several hours. Drain well and serve on bed of lettuce. Makes 4 servings.

Total recipe contains: 18 grams carbohydrate, 4 grams protein, and 0 grams fat.

One serving (½ cup) contains 5 grams carbohydrate, 1 gram protein, 0 fat, 25 calories, and vitamins A and C.

Exchange value: 1 serving = 1 Group A vegetable.

COMMENT: The mushrooms above are optional but must be fresh if used. Calculations remain as they are if mushrooms are omitted.

Salad Dressings

The usual varieties of tossed or mixed green salads are permissible as free foods. It is only when they are combined with high-fat dressings that trouble begins. Included below are a few recipes for low-calorie dressings that can indeed be considered free if reasonable amounts are used. Leafy green salads have much to recommend them nutritionally, and it is desirable that diabetics, as well as other members of the family, have generous servings daily.

The flavor of mayonnaise comes primarily from the lemon and herbs used in it. Oils used in commercial mayonnaise are generally flavorless, and therefore a variety of thickened mixtures appropriately flavored can pass as mayonnaise in a pinch. None of the dressings included here is as good as real mayonnaise, nor indeed have I ever tasted a substitute that was as good as the real thing. They will, however, suffice if you must have a very restricted fat intake, count calories, or simply find yourself at dinnertime with the day's allotment of fat used up and one meal left to go.

There are numerous kinds of packaged dressings that are quite flavorful. They are marketed under various trade names and sometimes have a special mixing bottle that can be purchased along with the dressing. The following combination can be used with any of the well-known brands available.

1 package salad dressing mix
2 tablespoons powdered pectin
3 tablespoons lemon juice
¾ cup water (or fill to the line marked "oil" if mixing kit is purchased)

These mixes contain negligible calories and nutrients but considerable flavor.

Occasionally I see a recipe for a "low-fat" or "reducing" mayonnaise that uses mineral oil as a base. Mineral oil is not absorbed and therefore would lend itself to low-fat diets; however, there are good nutritional reasons why this kind of oil should not be used. Salad greens contain large amounts of vitamin A, which will be lost along with the mineral oil. These greens may furnish the major part of vitamin A in the diet if it is extremely limited or if cooked greens are not eaten. Mineral oil mayonnaise cannot therefore be recommended.

LOW-FAT MAYONNAISE

1 can (13 ounces) evaporated
  skim milk
½ teaspoon unflavored gelatin
2 egg yolks
¾ teaspoon sugar

1½ teaspoons dry mustard
1 teaspoon salt
4 tablespoons fresh lemon juice
½ teaspoon lemon peel, grated

Reserve ¼ cup milk and sprinkle gelatin over the surface to soften. Heat remaining milk to scalding and add reserved portion containing gelatin. Remove from heat. Blend other ingredients (except lemon juice and peel) until smooth and add milk mixture, 3 to 4 tablespoons at a time. Blend well after each addition. When all milk has been added, transfer to double boiler and cook gently, stirring constantly until mixture coats the spoon. Remove and add lemon juice and peel. Mixture will thicken as it cools.

Total recipe contains: 43 grams carbohydrate, 34 grams protein, and 11 grams fat.

One tablespoon contains: 12 calories and may be used without counting any nutrient in the diabetic's diet.

CHEESE DRESSING

Combine the preceding mayonnaise with either Roquefort or blue cheese in the usual manner.

One tablespoon cheese contains: 3 grams protein, 4 grams fat, and 50 calories.

Exchange value: 1 tablespoon = 1 fat.

THOUSAND ISLAND DRESSING

1 small dill pickle, chopped
1 tablespoon catsup
1 tablespoon chopped parsley

½ cup Low-Fat Mayonnaise (see
  above)

Combine ingredients. Makes about ¾ cup.

Total recipe contains: 15 grams carbohydrate, 8 grams protein, and 3 grams fat.

One tablespoon contains: negligible amounts.

MAYONNAISE

½ teaspoon dry mustard
1 teaspoon salt
Juice of 1 lemon

1 egg
¾ cup safflower or other
   unsaturated oil

Put first four ingredients into a bowl and beat with a whisk until smooth. Add oil, 1 tablespoon at a time, for about five additions. Beat well after each addition. Pour remaining oil in a thin stream, beating constantly. Makes approximately 1 cup.

    Total recipe contains: 5 grams carbohydrate, 7 grams protein, and 156 grams fat.

    One teaspoon contains: 3 grams fat and 30 calories.

    Exchange value: 2 teaspoons = 1 fat.

FRESH HERB MAYONNAISE

Before beating mayonnaise (above) with whisk, add 2 tablespoons minced fresh parsley, 1 tablespoon minced fresh chives, and 2 teaspoons crumbled dry tarragon.

    Cut 1 head of Bibb lettuce into quarters, spread cut surface lightly with herb mayonnaise, and serve.

FRENCH DRESSING

4 tablespoons lemon juice
2 tablespoons powdered pectin
½ cup water

¾ teaspoon salt
¼ teaspoon paprika
1 tablespoon catsup

Combine ingredients. Shake well in a small jar and store in refrigerator.

    Total recipe contains: 7 grams carbohydrate and negligible amounts of nutrients and calories.

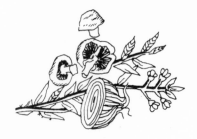

CHAPTER 7

Soups and Stocks

- Beef Stock
- Consommé
- Mushroom Consommé
- Onion Soup
- Zucchini Soup
- Spinach Beef Soup
- Chicken Stock
- Chicken Bouillon
- Chicken and Egg Soup

- Abalone Soup
- Chicken Cucumber Soup
- Chicken Mushroom Soup
- Tomato Squash Soup
- Fresh Pea Soup
- Cold Fresh Tomato Soup
- Mom's Vegetable Soup
- Spinach Soup

Many dishes included in this chapter contain few calories and only small amounts of carbohydrate. In most, not more than ½ fat exchange (2.5 grams) is present in a single serving. These dishes can be used to add bulk, vitamins, and minerals, especially in lower-calorie diets. Such diets are difficult to balance even for experienced nutritionists, and the low-calorie, low-fat, and low-carbohydrate recipes presented throughout this chapter should be used frequently to supplement regular meal plans.

Although it is possible to buy powders and cubes that make adequate meat stocks and bouillons, far more nutritious stocks can be made at home and stored if you have freezer space available. These are not inexpensive, but they are more flavorful as well as more nutritious than the commercial products. Probably most people will not prepare homemade stocks except for special dishes, since they do require more time than is needed for the commercially available mixes. However, since diabetics must be vigilant about nutrients, recipes for homemade meat stocks are included here. Commercial stocks can be substituted in all recipes.

The combination of meat stocks, vegetables, and fruits that make delicious, nutritious, low-calorie soups is limited only by the cook's imagination. Homemade stocks can make a valuable contribution, especially to diets of elderly people who may have poor teeth and poor appetites. These older folk often do not drink milk and consequently have little or no source of calcium and phosphorus. The stock-based soups provide an easily digestible source of these minerals, plus the small amount of protein that is usually needed. If commercial bouillon is used, add 2 tablespoons of plain gelatin to each quart of liquid to equal the protein content of the homemade product.

BEEF STOCK

3 pounds beef bones with some
  meat
3 quarts water
1 tablespoon vinegar
2½ teaspoons salt

1 green onion
1 tablespoon sherry
¼ teaspoon ginger
1 clove garlic
1 bay leaf

Brown bones slowly in heavy skillet or pot. When thoroughly brown on all sides, add other ingredients. Simmer 3 hours or so. Let cool. Strain stock into storage container and refrigerate or freeze. When chilled, skim off fat and discard. The stock should have the consistency of a heavy gelatin solution at this point.

COMMENT: Our dietitian says that browning the bones doesn't add much flavor and is a big bother. She recommends dumping the fresh bones directly into the water. Browning is recommended more for color than for flavor and can be omitted if color is not important for your purposes.

CONSOMMÉ

1 quart Beef Stock (above)
1 pinch each dried marjoram,
  thyme, and basil
1 small clove garlic, crushed and
  peeled

2 tablespoons chives, minced
1½ teaspoons salt

Simmer all ingredients 5 minutes. Strain into serving dishes and top with small amount of grated lemon rind or very thin slices of lemon.

One serving (1 cup) contains: 4 grams protein, 0 grams fat, 16 calories, calcium, phosphorus, and negligible carbohydrate.

This need not be counted on an exchange diet.

NUTRITION NOTE: Add 1 tablespoon (1 packet) of unflavored gelatin and increase the protein content by 7 grams (28 calories). A good mid-morning or afternoon snack!

MUSHROOM CONSOMMÉ

1 quart Beef Stock (page 70)   1½ teaspoons salt
½ pound mushrooms

Heat stock to a gentle simmer. Add mushrooms and simmer for 3 to 4 minutes. If canned mushrooms are used, add canning liquid as well, but heat only to serving temperature. Add salt to taste. Makes about 5 cups.

One serving (1 cup) contains: 4 grams protein, 16 calories, calcium, iron, B vitamins, and negligible carbohydrate and fat.

A 1-cup serving need not be counted on an exchange diet.

NUTRITION NOTE: Add 1 tablespoon (1 packet) unflavored gelatin and increase the protein content by 7 grams (28 calories). Another good snack!

ONION SOUP

1 quart Beef Stock (page 70)   1 tablespoon cooking sherry
1 teaspoon salt   Parmesan cheese
4 large onions, thinly sliced

Simmer stock and add salt, sliced onions, and sherry. Simmer 5 minutes. Strain and discard onions. Sprinkle with Parmesan cheese. Put under broiler until cheese becomes bubbly. Serve at once. Makes 4 cups.

Onions contain a significant amount of carbohydrate, and if left in must be counted in the daily intake. The above method gives considerable onion flavor without the added carbohydrate.

One serving (1 cup) contains: 4 grams protein, 16 calories, calcium, phosphorus, negligible carbohydrate, and no fat. It need not be counted in an exchange diet.

COMMENT: If you can afford the extra carbohydrate and wish to leave the onions in, count 10 grams of carbohydrate, 6 grams of protein, and 60 calories per cup.

ZUCCHINI SOUP

1 quart Beef Stock (page 70)   1 medium zucchini, diced
1½ teaspoons salt

Heat stock and add salt. Add zucchini and remove from heat. Keep tightly covered. Let sit for 5 minutes and serve. The zucchini should be quite crisp. Makes about 5 cups.

One serving (1 cup) contains: 2 grams carbohydrate, 4 grams protein, 0 grams fat, 25 calories, calcium, phosphorus, and vitamins A and C.

COMMENT: Zucchini quickly becomes mushy if overcooked. This can be prevented by applying the salt directly to the squash for a few minutes prior to cooking. Cooking must still be brief, however. Do not freeze this soup—the flavor of zucchini is altered by freezing.

SPINACH BEEF SOUP

1 large onion, quartered   1 bunch parsley, stemmed and
1 quart Beef Stock (page 70)   chopped
1 cup tomato purée
1 bunch spinach, stemmed and
   chopped

Add onion to stock and heat to boiling. Let cook for 3 to 4 minutes and remove onion. Add purée, shredded spinach, and parsley leaves. Let simmer for 1 minute. Serve immediately. Makes 5 to 6 cups. This delicious soup contains large amounts of vitamins A and B, calcium, phosphorus, and iron.

One serving (1 cup) contains: 4 grams carbohydrate, 4 grams protein, 0 grams fat, and 30 calories.

Exchange value: 1 cup = 1 vegetable exchange.

COMMENT: Cooking time must be carefully controlled for spinach soups. If cooked too long (2 minutes is usually too long), the spinach loses its consistency and the flavor is altered. Other greens, such as mustard, chard, and bok, can take slightly more cooking, but not much more. The temptation in the above recipe is to leave the onion in longer. To do so results in too much onion taste. If the onion is cooked in the soup for only 3 to 4 minutes, it is not identifiable as such.

CHICKEN STOCK

4 to 5 pounds chicken backs and
  necks
½ cup chopped onion
½ teaspoon dried thyme
Small bunch parsley

1 bay leaf
¼ teaspoon dried marjoram
3 quarts water
1½ teaspoons salt

Mix all ingredients and simmer for 3 to 4 hours. Strain into storage container and cool in refrigerator. Remove fat and save for flavoring other dishes. Freeze stock for use in soups and other dishes. The bones will be soft enough to use as pet food if you wish. Makes about 2 quarts stock.

COMMENT: If properly prepared, this stock should jell when refrigerated. It can therefore be used to prepare aspics or gelatin salads without the use of additional gelatin. The stock may not congeal after it has been frozen and so should be fresh when it is to be used in a gel. It is considerably more nutritious than the stock prepared from packaged gelatin and bouillon cubes.

One serving (1 cup) contains: 4 grams protein, negligible carbohydrate and fat, 16 calories, calcium, phosphorus, and B vitamins.

CHICKEN BOUILLON

1 quart Chicken Stock (above)
1½ teaspoons salt (or more,
  depending on stock)

Pinch dried sage

Mix ingredients, heat to serving temperature, and garnish with unpeeled red apple slices.

One serving (1 cup) contains: 3–4 grams protein, calcium, phosphorus, 16 calories, and negligible amounts of carbohydrate and fat.

Exchange value: It need not be counted on an exchange diet.

CHICKEN AND EGG SOUP

1 quart Chicken Stock (page 73)   1 egg, well beaten
1½ teaspoons salt   Chopped chives for garnish

Simmer stock and salt. Add beaten egg in a thin stream while stirring the soup quickly. Remove from heat and serve immediately. Garnish with chives.

One serving (1 cup) contains: 5 grams protein, 1 gram fat, 30 calories, calcium, iron, phosphorus, and small amounts of vitamins A and E.

Exchange value: It need not be counted on an exchange diet.

COMMENT: For low-fat diets, substitute 2 egg whites and a few drops of yellow food coloring for the whole egg. This eliminates the fat entirely and decreases the calories to 20 per serving. For higher-fat diets, add extra oil to individual servings. Increase fat count by 5 grams per teaspoon added and calories by 45 for each teaspoon added.

ABALONE SOUP

2 cups Chicken Stock (page 73)   ½ pound abalone
¼ pound fresh mushrooms   Salt to taste

Heat chicken stock to boiling; add mushrooms and abalone. Simmer 5 minutes. Add salt to taste. Serve with very thin lemon slices. Serves 4 as soup or 2 as a main course, accompanied by green salad and beverage.

Total recipe contains: 13 grams carbohydrate, 53 grams protein, negligible fat, and 270 calories.

One serving (¼ of total) contains: 3 grams carbohydrate, 13 grams protein, negligible fat, and 70 calories.

COMMENT: Scallops may be substituted if abalone is not available in your area.

CHICKEN CUCUMBER SOUP

1½ teaspoons salt
2 large cucumbers, diced

1 quart Chicken Stock (page 73)
Grated orange peel for garnish

Sprinkle salt over cucumbers and let stand for 15 minutes. Blot with paper towel. Simmer stock and add cucumbers. Turn off heat and let sit for 5 more minutes. Cucumbers should still be crisp. Garnish with grated orange peel. Makes 5 to 6 cups.

One serving (1 cup) contains: 4 grams protein, 0 grams fat, and 16 calories.

Exchange value: It need not be counted on an exchange diet.

CHICKEN MUSHROOM SOUP

1 quart Chicken Stock (page 73)
1½ teaspoons salt

½ pound fresh or canned
  mushrooms

Simmer stock and add salt and mushrooms. Simmer 4 to 5 minutes and serve. If canned mushrooms are used, add liquid and heat only to serving temperature. Makes 5 cups.

One serving (1 cup) contains: 4 grams protein, 16 calories, calcium, and phosphorus.

Exchange value: It need not be counted on an exchange diet.

TOMATO SQUASH SOUP

2 cups tomatoes (preferably fresh),
  peeled and chopped
½ cup diced yellow squash

¼ teaspoon dill
Salt to taste

Combine ingredients. Simmer 5 to 8 minutes (squash should still be crisp). Add salt to taste. Makes four servings of ½ cup each.

One serving (½ cup) contains: 5 grams carbohydrate, 1 gram protein, 25 calories, and vitamins A, B, and C.

Exchange value: 1 Group A vegetable.

FRESH PEA SOUP

1 cup fresh peas (cooked in 1 cup water or Chicken Stock, page 73)	1 teaspoon sugar
	½ teaspoon MSG
	Nutmeg
2 cups half and half	Salt to taste

Put peas, including any liquid left from cooking, into blender. Blend until smooth. Add a little of the half and half if necessary to get a smooth consistency. Add all remaining ingredients except nutmeg and salt. Warm in top of double boiler until steaming but not boiling. Add salt to taste (it won't take much). Transfer to serving dishes. Sprinkle each dish with just a whisper of nutmeg. Serves 4 to 6.

Total recipe contains: 44 grams carbohydrate, 23 grams protein, 57 grams fat, and 766 calories.

One serving (⅙ of total) contains: 7 grams carbohydrate, 4 grams protein, 9 grams fat, and 128 calories.

Exchange value: 1 serving = ½ bread and 2 fat.

COMMENT: My introduction to this treatment of pea soup was in Perino's Restaurant in Los Angeles. It was the first course of a marvelous luncheon that included cold poached salmon and cucumbers with sour cream, lightly seasoned with fresh dill. I highly recommend the combination to you.

COLD FRESH TOMATO SOUP

6 large tomatoes, peeled and coarsely chopped	½ teaspoon salt
	¼ cup Mayonnaise (page 68)
1 large sweet white onion, chopped	2 teaspoons curry powder
	Parsley, finely chopped, for
½ teaspoon MSG	garnish

Put tomatoes, onion, MSG, and salt into the food processor. Chop until onion is finely chopped but tomatoes still have a few chunks intact. Chill well. Mix mayonnaise and curry and chill. Serve in chilled cups and garnish with a dollop of mayonnaise and a sprinkle of parsley. For good flavor, this requires excellent fully ripened tomatoes. It makes a good introduction to a Spanish or Mexican meal. Serves 6.

Total recipe contains: 67 grams carbohydrate, 16 grams protein, and 48 grams fat.

One serving (⅙ of total) contains: 11 grams carbohydrate, 3 grams protein, 8 grams fat, and 128 calories.

Exchange value: 1 serving = 2 vegetable and 1½ fat.

LOW-FAT NOTE: This recipe can be adapted to a low-fat diet by substituting Low-Fat Mayonnaise (page 67). In that case subtract all of the fat and reduce the calories in 1 serving to 56.

MOM'S VEGETABLE SOUP
(Or Make-It-out-of-What-You've-Got Soup)

1 pork bone (a ham hock is great but a pork chop bone will do)
Salt and pepper to taste
2 tablespoons bacon fat (if using pork chop bone)
2 large, very ripe tomatoes
½ cup fresh lima beans

½ cup green peas
½ cup yellow squash
½ cup green beans
1 cup fresh corn
1 cup okra, sliced crosswise
1 clove garlic, grated
1 bay leaf

If you're using a pork chop bone, salt it well and brown lightly in the bacon fat. Discard the fat. If you're using a ham hock, just put everything in the pot and simmer gently until some juice begins to form. Stir only to prevent sticking. Taste occasionally for salt and pepper and doneness. Serve this with hot corn bread, a big slice of sharp cheddar cheese, and a glass of buttermilk on a crisp fall day. Serves 8.

Total recipe contains: 82 grams carbohydrate, 21 grams protein, and 17 grams fat.

One serving (⅛ of total) contains: 10 grams carbohydrate, 3 grams protein, 2 grams fat, and 70 calories.

COMMENT: Actually, my mother has never made soup by this recipe, because the ingredients in her soup have never been the same twice. She and my father have always cultivated a garden that, in a reasonable year, might feed a community of a thousand.

This soup was usually made from the odds and ends of the late fall garden or from ½ cup of lots of things put in the freezer or canned for later use. It is a generous soup that will suffer dozens of amendments without any loss in palatability.

SPINACH SOUP

1 quart water or Chicken Stock   1 teaspoon salt
    (page 73)   ¼ teaspoon sugar
2 bunches (about ½ pound)   ½ teaspoon MSG
    spinach, stemmed and shredded   2 teaspoons sesame oil

Bring water to boiling and add greens (chard, mustard, or turnip greens
can be used, but spinach is very good), salt, sugar, and MSG. Boil 2
minutes. Remove from heat. Add ½ teaspoon sesame oil to *each* serving. Serves 4.

One serving (1 cup) contains: 3 grams fat, vitamins A, B, and C, and
35 calories.

Exchange value: 1 cup = ½ fat exchange + 1 Group A vegetable
exchange.

COMMENT: If your diet requires larger amounts of fat, this soup can
easily accommodate more than is recommended above. Each cup can
carry 1 to 2 teaspoons. Don't forget to allow for the extra and to include
the extra fat exchanges if you add more.

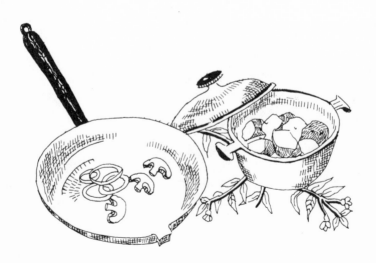

CHAPTER 8

Meat, Fish, Fowl, and Eggs

- Crab Cakes
- Crab Pilaf
- Crab-Stuffed Onions
- Crab Marinade
- Grilled Shrimp
- Shrimp with Green Beans
- Shrimp and Wild Rice
- Pinkie's Shrimp Creole
- Curried Shrimp
- Scallops Almondine
- Vegetarian Prawns
- Broiled Scallops
- Baked Oysters
- Oyster Roast
- Hangtown Fry
- Serendipity Trout
- Tuna and Vegetables
- Tuna Pie
- Tuna Salad
- Smoke-Flavored Halibut
- Fish Stew
- Brennan's Swordfish
- Cioppino
- Smothered Fish
- Creole Halibut
- Salmon Steaks with Dressing

- Grilled Salmon
- Smoked Salmon Steaks
- Smoked Turkey Roast
- Chicken Little
- East Indian Chicken
- Chicken Breasts with Orange Sauce
- Mint Chicken
- Smoked Chicken
- Hannah Spielholz's Chicken
- Oven-Fried Chicken
- Chicken with Peanuts
- Chicken Divan, Brennan's Way
- Skip Schmidt's Tumwater Chicken
- Angela's Pheasant
- Sweet and Sour Pork
- Spiced Pork and Veal
- Barbecued Pork
- Katie's Persian Lamb
- Epicurean Lamb
- Lamb and Spring Onions
- Ground Beef with Butter Beans
- Beef Spinach Scramble
- Ginger Beef with Little Green Onions

79

- **Beef with Broccoli**
- **Beef Wine Stew**
- **Tomato Meat Loaf**
- **Roasted Soybeans**
- **Eggs with Scallops**

- **Egg Flower Soup**
- **Quiche Lorraine**
- **Scrambled Eggs**
- **Fancy Scrambled Eggs**

CRAB CAKES

1 slice white bread
2 eggs, beaten
½ teaspoon salt
1½ teaspoons dry mustard
½ stick butter or margarine,
    melted

1 tablespoon finely chopped
    parsley
1 pound crab meat

Tear the bread into very small pieces and add to beaten eggs. Add remaining ingredients to crab and mix well. Add egg-and-bread mixture. This should be quite thick, the consistency of heavy dough. Form into 12 cakes, place on a cookie sheet, and refrigerate until quite firm.

Brown in a heavy iron skillet or a nonstick heavy pan. Don't overcrowd. There will be enough fat in cakes to prevent sticking.

These can be prepared ahead and rewarmed just before serving. They may be even better this way. Serves 6 generously.

Total recipe contains: 15 grams carbohydrate, 95 grams protein, and 67 grams fat.

One serving (2 cakes) contains: 3 grams carbohydrate, 16 grams protein, and 11 grams fat.

Exchange value: 1 serving = 2 medium-fat meats.

CRAB PILAF

1 medium onion, sliced
1 tablespoon unsaturated
    margarine
1 pound cooked crab meat
1 can (10½ ounces) tomato soup

½ teaspoon salt
¼ teaspoon pepper
1 teaspoon dry mint

Sauté the onion in the margarine until clear. Add remaining ingredients and simmer 5 to 6 minutes. Serve with steamed rice (allow ½ cup rice per serving). There should be about three cups total. Serves 4.

Total recipe contains: 45 grams carbohydrate, 86 grams protein, and 26 grams fat.

One serving (¼ of total with ½ cup rice) contains: 30 grams carbohydrate, 24 grams protein, 7 grams fat, and 230 calories.

COMMENT: Serve this with a tossed green salad, without additional bread unless your carbohydrate allowance is generous. The dish can be prepared in advance by mixing all ingredients except the crab. The sauce actually improves with some age. It can be quickly heated and the crab added at the last minute for a quick meal.

Exchange value: ½ cup rice = 1 bread; ¼ of crab mixture = 3 lean meat + 1 bread.

Since the crab has such a low fat content, it may be necessary to include another fat exchange (5 grams) elsewhere in the meal. Although the protein content is equivalent to three meat exchanges, the fat content is not.

This is very nice for those counting calories.

CRAB-STUFFED ONIONS

4 large onions	¼ teaspoon curry powder
1½ cups cooked crab meat	1 tablespoon Mayonnaise (page 68)
¾ cups minced celery	
¼ cup minced green pepper	⅛ teaspoon Tabasco

Parboil whole onions in salted water for about 10 to 15 minutes. Remove all inner layers and use for another dish, leaving outermost one or two layers intact. Mix remaining ingredients and fill onions. Chill.

Total recipe contains: 17 grams carbohydrate, 47 grams protein, and 17 grams fat.

One serving (¼ of total) contains: 4 grams carbohydrate, 12 grams protein, 4 grams fat, and about 100 calories.

Exchange value: ¼ of total recipe (1 onion) = 2 meat + 1 Group A vegetable.

COMMENT: If the onion is not eaten, deduct 4 grams of carbohydrate and 15 calories.

CRAB MARINADE

1 pound cooked crab meat
¼ cup lemon juice
¼ cup oil
½ cup dry white wine
1 clove garlic, grated

1 teaspoon salt
⅛ teaspoon Tabasco
1 egg, beaten
Lettuce leaves

Toss crab with lemon juice. Combine all ingredients except lettuce and add to crab. Marinate for at least 1 hour or overnight in refrigerator. Drain and serve on a lettuce leaf.

Total recipe contains: 12 grams carbohydrate, 85 grams protein, 64 grams fat, and 10 grams alcohol.

One serving (3 ounces) contains: 15 grams protein, 3 grams fat, and 90 calories.

Exchange value: 1 serving = 2 meat.

COMMENT: This can also be served warm on a bed of rice.

GRILLED SHRIMP

1 package instant meat marinade
½ teaspoon basil
½ teaspoon tarragon

½ teaspoon celery seed
2 pounds shrimp or prawns

Dilute instant marinade according to directions on package and add herbs. Butterfly shrimp and dip in marinade. Barbecue immediately over coals or in oven. Baste with marinade as they cook. They should be done in about 5 minutes. Serves 6.

One ounce contains: 5 grams protein, 1 gram fat, and 30 calories.
Exchange value: 3 ounces (1 serving) = 2 meat.

COMMENT: These can be quickly prepared. The marinade can be made anytime and refrigerated. The shrimp can be swirled in the marinade and put in a strainer to drain while some are cooking. They make elegant party snacks or a tasty main dish served with rice or other vegetable and a salad.

SHRIMP WITH GREEN BEANS

1 tablespoon oil	1 pound raw shrimp
2 pounds green beans, diagonally sliced	⅛ teaspoon pepper
	¼ cup chicken bouillon
½ teaspoon salt	1 tablespoon soy sauce

Heat oil to very hot in heavy pan; add beans and salt. Stir-fry about 4 minutes. Remove beans and stir-fry shrimp in same pan about 2 minutes. Add beans and other ingredients. Cover and steam for about 5 more minutes. Serves 4.

Entire recipe contains: 58 grams carbohydrate, 98 grams protein, and 19 grams fat.

One serving (3 ounces) contains: 14 grams carbohydrate, 25 grams protein, 5 grams of fat, and 200 calories.

Exchange value: 3 ounces (1 serving) = 3 lean meat + 2 vegetable.

COMMENT: Prawns may be substituted for shrimp without changing calculations.

SHRIMP AND WILD RICE

1 onion, chopped	½ teaspoon salt
1 tablespoon unsaturated margarine	½ teaspoon tarragon
	½ teaspoon garlic salt
1 pound fresh mushrooms	½ pound crab meat
2 tablespoons lemon juice	2 cups cooked wild rice
1 pound shrimp	Green onions or parsley, chopped, for garnish
¼ cup Chicken Stock (page 73)	
¼ cup dry white cooking wine	

Sauté onion in margarine; add mushrooms and lemon juice. Cook gently 2 to 3 minutes. Add shrimp and continue sautéing until shrimp turn pink. Add remaining ingredients except rice and garnish and simmer 2 to 3 minutes. Combine with cooked wild rice and let sit for a few minutes until flavors have time to mix. Garnish with tops of chopped green onions or chopped parsley. Serves 6.

Total recipe contains: 39 grams carbohydrate, 136 grams protein, and 19 grams fat.

One serving (⅙ of total and ⅓ cup rice) contains: 22 grams carbohydrate, 25 grams protein, 3 grams fat, and 115 calories.

Exchange value: 1 serving (⅙ of total and ⅓ cup rice) = 1 vegetable, 3 lean meat, and 1 bread.

COMMENT: There are many pitfalls in calculating a mixed recipe such as the foregoing, and this has made those of us who work with diabetics leery of recommending mixed dishes or casseroles. When I say you can obtain the content of one serving by dividing the total content by the number of servings, I assume that the servings are equal. This is often not the case. If you are feeding small children or a mixed group, the servings may well differ in size. To calculate accurately, the portion to be measured must first be removed. Thus, if you are serving the foregoing recipe to six people and wish to measure only one portion, you can proceed as follows:

1. Measure wild rice into small casserole dish or serving dish.
2. Measure total volume of shrimp mixture.
3. Remove ⅙ (or whatever fraction) and add to wild rice in serving dish; cover and let flavors blend.
4. Serve remainder in usual way to the other diners.

PINKIE'S SHRIMP CREOLE

2 medium onions, chopped	⅓ teaspoon celery salt
1 medium green pepper, chopped	¼ teaspoon thyme
1 clove garlic	2 teaspoons minced parsley
2 teaspoons oil	1 pound cooked shrimp
2 tablespoons flour	2 tablespoons Worcestershire
1 large can (2½ cups) tomatoes	sauce
2 bay leaves	Salt to taste

Add onion, pepper, and garlic to oil in skillet and sauté 4 to 5 minutes. Blend in flour. Add tomatoes and seasoning. Simmer 30 minutes. Add shrimp and Worcestershire sauce and cook 15 minutes longer. Salt to taste. Serve on rice. Serves 4.

Total recipe contains: 59 grams carbohydrate, 92 grams protein, and 14 grams fat.

One serving (¼ total amount of creole) contains: 15 grams carbohydrate, 23 grams protein, 4 grams fat, and 190 calories.

Exchange value: ¼ total recipe = 1 Group B vegetable, ½ bread, and 3 meat.

CURRIED SHRIMP

1 pound shrimp, shelled and
  deveined
¼ cup unsaturated margarine
1 medium onion, finely chopped
⅛ teaspoon powdered ginger

1 tablespoon curry powder
2 tablespoons flour
1¼ cups skim milk
1 teaspoon salt

Sauté shrimp in the margarine until they change color. Remove and keep warm. Add onion, ginger, and curry; cook until onion is clear. Add flour and stir until smooth. Add milk and stir until well mixed. Add salt and shrimp. Do not boil. Serves 6.

Total recipe contains: 42 grams carbohydrate, 96 grams protein, and 49 grams fat.

Each serving (⅙ of total) contains: 7 grams carbohydrate, 16 grams protein, 8 grams fat, and 100 calories.

Exchange value: ⅙ of total = 2 lean meat and ½ bread.

SCALLOPS ALMONDINE

1 pound scallops
Paprika
2 tablespoons lemon juice

4 teaspoons margarine
¼ cup chopped almonds
½ teaspoon salt

Sprinkle scallops generously with paprika, then lemon juice. Melt margarine in metal baking dish and add almonds and scallops. Sprinkle salt over all. Bake in 350° oven for 15 minutes. The scallops will cook quickly. Serves 4.

Total recipe contains: 25 grams carbohydrate, 76 grams protein, 36 grams fat, and 740 calories.

One serving (¼ of total) contains: 6 grams carbohydrate, 20 grams protein, 9 grams fat, and 185 calories.

Exchange value: 1 serving = 3 meat and 1 Group A vegetable.

COMMENT: Unless all the sauce is eaten, the fat estimate given above is a little high. If you wish to take this into consideration, drain the scallops after cooking and measure the fat retrieved. The discarded fat can be substracted from the total. This dish is good served with clam nectar, sliced tomatoes, and asparagus tips.

VEGETARIAN PRAWNS

1½ cups cooked mashed potatoes 1 tablespoon sherry
¼ cup soy flour   1 teaspoon salt
1 grated carrot   1 teaspoon MSG
1 tablespoon cornstarch   Oil for deep frying
2 egg whites

Mix all ingredients well. Shape into prawnlike balls. Deep-fry until brown. Serve with hot mustard or Chinese red sauce dip. Serves 4.

Total recipe contains: 61 grams carbohydrate, 21 grams protein, 17 grams fat, and 2 grams alcohol.

One serving (¼ of total) contains: 15 grams carbohydrate, 5 grams protein, 4 grams fat, and 116 calories.

Exchange value: 1 serving = 1 bread and 2 fat (includes fat used in frying).

BROILED SCALLOPS

1 teaspoon corn oil   ⅓ cup skim milk
1 pound scallops   ¼ teaspoon paprika
4 teaspoons lemon juice

Use oil to grease pan. Toss scallops with lemon juice; then dip in milk. Place in greased pan and sprinkle with paprika. Oven-broil until brown. Turn when necessary. Serves 4.

Total recipe contains: 20 grams carbohydrate, 72 grams protein, 6 grams fat, and 440 calories.

One serving (3 ounces) contains: 18 grams protein, 3 grams fat, and 110 calories.

Exchange value: 1 serving (3 ounces) = 2 lean meat.

BAKED OYSTERS

1 pound oysters   Onion flakes ·
Garlic salt   Parmesan cheese
Black pepper

Leave oysters in the half shell or put in individual serving dishes. Weigh or measure diabetic's portion before cooking. Sprinkle each serving with garlic salt, black pepper, onion flakes, and Parmesan cheese (not more than 1 teaspoon per serving). Bake in slow oven 30 minutes or until oysters curl around the edges. Serves 4.

Total recipe contains: 30 grams carbohydrate, 58 grams protein, and 17 grams fat.

One serving (¼ of total recipe) contains: 7.5 grams carbohydrate, 14.5 grams protein, 4 grams fat, and 85 calories.

Exchange value: 1 serving (¼ of total) = 1 lean meat + ½ bread.

OYSTER ROAST

4 ounces oysters (¼ pint)
1 tablespoon lemon juice
1 tablespoon butter or margarine
¼ cup coarse cracker crumbs
2 teaspoons sherry

1 tablespoon cream
1 teaspoon Worcestershire sauce
Dash tabasco
Pinch salt
Pinch garlic powder

Sprinkle oysters with lemon juice. Melt butter in an individual serving dish and sprinkle cracker crumbs over bottom of dish. Add the oysters in a single layer. Take any liquor remaining from oysters and add to it the remaining ingredients. Drizzle over the oysters and bake at 425° for 15 minutes. Serves 1.

One serving (total recipe) contains: 23 grams carbohydrate, 15 grams protein, 18 grams fat, 2 grams alcohol, and 324 calories.

Exchange value: 1½ bread, 2 medium-fat meat, and 2 fat.

HANGTOWN FRY

2 medium oysters (about 2 ounces)
1 cup lightly salted boiling water
Scant ½ teaspoon bacon
   drippings

2 eggs, beaten lightly
⅛ teaspoon Tabasco
1 green onion, chopped
1 slice cooked bacon, crumbled

Add oysters to boiling water for 1 minute. Remove, drain, and chop into bite-size pieces. Heat an omelet pan moderately hot and add the bacon drippings. Combine eggs and Tabasco and add to omelet pan. When lightly set, add oysters, green onion (reserving a few green pieces for garnish), and bacon. Fold the omelet over and serve on a warm plate. Serves 1.

(continued)

Total recipe contains: 7 grams carbohydrate, 21 grams protein, 17 grams fat, and 261 calories.

Exchange value: 3 medium-fat meat and 1 vegetable.

COMMENT: This is a good Sunday brunch served with hot biscuits.

SERENDIPITY TROUT

Trout   2 teaspoons garlic-flavored oil
Celery salt   Plastic baking bag
Instant chicken bouillon granules

Wash trout, or other fish, and sprinkle inside of cavity with celery salt and the chicken bouillon powder. Dry the outside of the fish and coat with small amount of cooking oil. Place inside the plastic baking bag, seal, and put on *top* rack of your dishwasher. Run the dishwasher through a full cycle.

Your fish will be deliciously done at the end of the cycle. If you're in the mood to socialize a bit more, it will hold nicely without overcooking for another half hour. Serves 4.

Total recipe with 1 pound rainbow or steelhead trout, dressed, contains: 98 grams protein and 62 grams fat.

One 4-ounce serving contains: 24 grams protein, 15 grams fat, and 236 calories.

Exchange value: 1 serving (4 ounces) = 3½ lean meat and 1 fat.

Total recipe with 1 pound brook trout, dressed, contains: 87 grams protein, and 20 grams fat.

One serving (4 ounces) contains: 22 grams protein, 5 grams fat, and 121 calories.

Exchange value: 1 serving (4 ounces) = 3 lean meat.

TUNA AND VEGETABLES

¼ cup oil or margarine   1 can (5 ounces) bamboo shoots
1 cup thinly sliced carrots   ¼ teaspoon salt
1 cup diagonally sliced green   ⅓ cup dry sherry
  onions   ½ cup chicken bouillon
1 cup diagonally sliced celery   1 cup raw spinach, shredded
2 cans (7 ounces each)   ¼ cup soy sauce
  water-packed tuna

Heat oil in heavy pan; add carrots, onion, and celery and stir-fry for 3 to 4 minutes. Add tuna, bamboo shoots, salt, sherry, and bouillon. Simmer 2 minutes and add spinach and soy sauce. Turn off heat, cover, and let set 2 to 3 minutes. Serve on steamed rice with pan sauce over the rice. Makes about 6 one-cup servings.

Total recipe contains: 49 grams carbohydrate, 121 grams protein, 54 grams fat, and 1116 calories.

One serving (⅙ total weight) contains: 8 grams carbohydrate, 20 grams protein, 9 grams of fat, and 145 calories

Exchange value: 1 serving (1 cup) = 3 meat and 1 Group B vegetable.

COMMENT: To adapt for low-fat diets, reduce amount of fat to 1 tablespoon. The entire recipe then contains 17 grams of fat, and one serving contains 2 to 3 grams fat and about 130 calories.

TUNA PIE

Pie Crust (page 90)
⅔ cup chopped onion
⅓ cup chopped green pepper
1 clove garlic, chopped
2 tablespoons chopped parsley
1 teaspoon basil

⅛ teaspoon pepper
½ teaspoon salt
2 cans (9¼ ounces each) water-packed tuna
1 large tomato, thinly sliced

Line pie pan with bottom crust. Combine onion, green pepper, garlic, parsley, basil, pepper, and salt and cover bottom of crust with about one-half mixture. Add a layer of tuna and a layer of tomato slices. Repeat until all ingredients are used. Make at least two layers. Cover with remaining pie crust. Bake in 400° oven for 35 minutes. Cut pie into 6 equal servings.

Total recipe contains: 106 grams carbohydrate, 193 grams protein, 108 grams fat, and 2160 calories.

Each slice contains: 18 grams carbohydrate, 32 grams protein, 18 grams fat, and 360 calories.

Exchange value: 1 bread, 5 meat, and 1 Group A vegetable.

To adapt for a low-fat diet: Omit the pie crust.

Total recipe then contains: 21 grams carbohydrate, 150 grams protein, and 4 grams fat.

A single serving contains: 4 grams carbohydrate, 24 grams protein, 1 gram fat, and 130 calories.

Exchange value: 3 meat and 1 Group A vegetable.

(continued)

COMMENT: It is not always possible to find water-packed tuna. If your grocer doesn't stock it, ask him to order some for you.

Pie Crust

½ cup unsaturated margarine, frozen
⅛ teaspoon salt

¾ cup white flour
¾ cup soy flour
2 egg whites, unbeaten

Using a fork, blend margarine, salt, and flours until the crumbles are about the size of small peas. Add egg whites and hand-mold mixture into halves. Roll out on a lightly floured board and fit bottom crust into a pan.

TUNA SALAD

2 tomatoes, cut in wedges
⅓ cup toasted sliced almonds
Shredded lettuce
1 cup shredded carrots
1 cup shredded zucchini
1 can (7 ounces) water-packed tuna

1 tablespoon chopped pickle
1 teaspoon celery seed
1 tablespoon lemon juice
⅓ cup Low-Fat Mayonnaise (page 67)

Reserve tomatoes, almonds, and lettuce. Mix other ingredients until well blended. Arrange salad on beds of shredded lettuce; add tomato wedges and garnish with toasted almonds. Serves 6.

Total recipe contains: 53 grams carbohydrate, 77 grams protein, 31 grams fat, and vitamins A, B, and C.

One serving (⅔ cup) contains: 9 grams carbohydrate, 13 grams protein, 5 grams fat, and 135 calories.

Exchange value: 1 serving (⅔ cup) = 2 meat and 1 Group B vegetable.

COMMENT: Serve with a hearty vegetable soup and milk to make a complete meal. A weight watcher might combine with a clear soup and skim milk for a nutritious and relatively low-calorie meal.

SMOKE-FLAVORED HALIBUT

2 pounds halibut steaks
⅓ cup soy sauce
2 tablespoons sherry

⅓ teaspoon liquid smoke flavoring
½ teaspoon ginger root, grated
1 tablespoon hoisin sauce

Combine all ingredients in a plastic bag and marinate 1 hour or longer in the refrigerator. Remove fish from plastic bag to covered dish, discard marinade, and bake fish in 250° oven for 20 minutes or until it flakes easily. Serve with green vegetable and corn bread. Serves 6.

Total recipe contains: 11 grams carbohydrate, 190 grams protein, and 11 grams fat.

One serving (4 ounces) contains: 30 grams protein, 2 grams fat, and 140 calories.

Exchange value: 1 serving = 3 lean meat.

FISH STEW

1 small onion, finely chopped	1 bay leaf
1 tablespoon oil	½ cup Chicken Stock (page 73)
¼ teaspoon garlic salt	or canned chicken broth
1 can (1 pound) whole tomatoes	2 stalks celery, whole
1 can (6 ounces) tomato paste	¼ teaspoon salt
1 bunch parsley	⅛ teaspoon Tabasco
½ teaspoon basil	2 pounds deboned fish, any kind
½ teaspoon oregano	

Sauté onion in oil until clear. Add everything except fish and simmer for 1 to 2 hours. Cube fish and add to sauce. Turn off heat and let sit in sauce for 10 to 15 minutes. Longer cooking results in a fishy taste. Remove parsley, celery, and bay leaf if you can find it. Serve in large soup plates with sourdough bread and green salad. Serves 6 generously.

Total recipe contains: 46 grams carbohydrate, 191 grams protein, and 25 grams fat.

One serving (⅙ of total) contains: 7 grams carbohydrate, 32 grams protein, and 4 grams fat.

Leftover (or fresh) chicken can be substituted without changing the calculations. This dish makes a good vehicle for combined leftovers.

Exchange value: 1 serving (⅙ of total) = 4 meat (see COMMENT).

COMMENT: Since a generous serving of this stew contains 32 grams of protein (4 meat exchanges) but only 4 grams of fat (instead of the 20 grams of fat assumed in the exchange list for 4 meat exchanges), 16 grams of fat (20 minus 4) are "saved" and can be used for butter on the French bread that is such a good accompaniment to this dish or for a rich salad dressing. When you wish to use rich sauces or salad dressings, always combine them with dishes such as this, and never with meats that are already high in fat content, and saturated fat at that.

BRENNAN'S SWORDFISH

1½ pounds swordfish, cubed   ⅛ teaspoon Tabasco
1½ cups white vinegar   1 bay leaf
½ cup water   1½ teaspoons salt
2 cloves garlic, crushed

Combine all ingredients and marinate several hours. Drain off marinade and broil fish until well done. Serves 6.

Total recipe contains: 15 grams carbohydrate, 130 grams protein, 27 grams fat, and 300 calories.

One serving (4 ounces) contains: 32 grams protein, 8 grams fat, and 50 calories.

Exchange value: 1 serving (4 ounces) = 4 low-fat meat.

CIOPPINO

1 can (1 pound, 12 ounces)   1 tablespoon lemon juice
  tomatoes   1 bunch parsley
1 can (8 ounces) tomato purée   1¼ cups Chicken Stock (page 73)
1 large green pepper, chopped   or 1 can (10½ ounces)
1 medium onion, chopped   condensed chicken broth
1 clove garlic   Salt to taste
1 bay leaf   1 pound fish, deboned
1 teaspoon sugar   1 pound shrimp
¼ teaspoon black pepper   1 dozen clams, in shell
⅛ teaspoon thyme   ½ pound crab meat

Combine tomatoes and all remaining ingredients except fish and shellfish. Simmer 10 minutes. Adjust seasoning. Layer fish and shellfish in a deep baking dish. Cover with sauce and simmer at least 20 minutes. Serve in large soup plates with green salad and sourdough bread. Serves 6 generously. There should be about 6 cups of sauce.

Total recipe contains: 87 grams carbohydrate, 269 grams protein, and 18 grams fat.

One serving of sauce (⅙ of total sauce) contains: 15 grams carbohydrate.

Exchange value: 1 serving of sauce = 1 bread.

One serving (3 ounces) of fish contains: 21 grams protein, 6 grams fat, and 150 calories.

Exchange value: 1 serving (3 ounces) of fish = 3 meat.

COMMENT: Any combination of fish and shellfish can be used in this dish. The flavor is improved if the shells are left on during cooking, but this does not add to the ease of eating. Shells may also complicate the weighing process if the meal must be weighed.

SMOTHERED FISH

Few drops oil
2 pounds fish, white
1 teaspoon granular chicken concentrate

1 tablespoon ginger root, sliced
4 mushrooms, chopped
1 green onion, chopped
2 tablespoons soy sauce

Oil bottom of glass baking dish and place fish on bottom. Sprinkle chicken concentrate over fish; add sliced ginger root, chopped mushrooms, green onion, and soy sauce. Cover and bake in slow oven (about 250 degrees) for 15 to 20 minutes. Serves 6.

Total recipe contains: 10 grams carbohydrate, 182 grams protein, 10 grams fat, and 840 calories.

One serving (⅙ of total) contains: 30 grams protein, 2 grams fat, and 140 calories.

Exchange value: 1 serving = 3 lean meat.

CREOLE HALIBUT

2 pounds fresh halibut
1 tablespoon minced onion
½ green pepper, minced

¼ teaspoon pepper
1 bay leaf, crumbled
2 cups canned tomatoes

Simmer ingredients in skillet for approximately 15 to 20 minutes. Makes 6 servings.

Total recipe contains: 20 grams carbohydrate, 179 grams protein, 10 grams fat, and 930 calories.

One serving (⅙ of total) contains: 3 grams carbohydrate, 29 grams protein, 3 grams fat, and 155 calories.

Exchange value: 1 serving = 4 meat and 1 Group A vegetable.

COMMENT: Any white fish may be substituted for halibut in this recipe.

SALMON STEAKS WITH DRESSING

¼ cup unsaturated margarine
4 salmon steaks, about 4–5
   ounces each
1 small onion, chopped
1 cup coarse bread crumbs

½ teaspoon salt
¼ teaspoon ground allspice
¼ teaspoon black pepper
¼ cup grapefruit juice
Grapefruit sections for garnish

Coat bottom of small baking dish with some of the margarine. Place steaks on bottom of baking dish. Sauté onion in remainder of margarine and add bread crumbs, salt, allspice, and pepper. Pour grapefruit juice over steaks and put the bread crumb mixture in the cavity of each steak. Place a grapefruit section on each mound of dressing. Bake in 350° oven for 10 minutes or until dressing is fairly dry and fish flakes easily. Serves 4.

One serving (¼ of total) contains: 15 grams carbohydrate, 20 grams protein, 25 grams fat, and 230 calories.

Exchange value: 1 serving (¼ of total) = 1 bread, 2 medium-fat meat, and 2 fat.

GRILLED SALMON

¼ teaspoon garlic salt
1 teaspoon lime juice
¼ cup soy sauce

4 salmon steaks, about 4 ounces
   each

Mix garlic salt, lime juice, and soy sauce and marinate steaks in mixture for 1 hour. Drain off marinade and broil steaks about 10 minutes on each side. If oven broiler is used, place broiler in lowest position. Weigh each portion of steak.

Each steak contains: 20 grams protein, 16 grams fat, and 222 calories.

Exchange value: 1 serving = 3 medium-fat meat.

COMMENT: If fresh salmon steaks are not available in your area, try swordfish. Swordfish is somewhat drier but still quite tasty. The calculations are interchangeable. Salmon just happened to be available when the recipe was tested.

SMOKED SALMON STEAKS

¼ cup soy sauce
2 tablespoons sherry or 1 tablespoon lime juice
½ teaspoon smoke flavoring

½ teaspoon grated ginger root or ¼ teaspoon powdered ginger
1 tablespoon hoisin sauce
4 salmon steaks, 4 ounces each

Combine all ingredients except salmon steaks. Marinate steaks in mixture for at least 1 hour. Remove from marinade, place on rack, and bake in 325° oven for 20 to 30 minutes or until fish flakes easily.

Each steak contains: 20 grams protein, 16 grams fat, and 222 calories.

Exchange value: 1 serving (1 steak) = 3 medium-fat meat.

COMMENT: The ginger root and hoisin sauce can be purchased in Oriental markets or in the specialty-food sections of many large supermarkets. Powdered ginger is not nearly so flavorful as the grated ginger root but is better than no ginger at all. There is no substitute for the hoisin sauce. This is usually sold in a small tin. Remove the total contents after opening and store in a tightly covered refrigerator jar. It will keep for several months. Hoisin sauce is composed of soybeans, brown beans, and spices. Some brands also list sugar as an ingredient. Since the sauce is always used in small quantities as a marinade, this need not be included in calculations.

SMOKED TURKEY ROAST

2½ pounds boneless turkey roast
2 tablespoons liquid smoke flavoring

1 teaspoon dried thyme
⅛ teaspoon cayenne
1 tablespoon lemon juice

Mix all ingredients in a plastic bag big enough to hold the turkey roast. Wrap bag around the roast and remove the air. All surfaces of the roast should be covered with the marinade. Put in the refrigerator and leave overnight or for several hours. Remove plastic bag and bake turkey according to directions on the package.

One ounce contains: 7 grams protein, 3 grams fat, and 50 calories.
Exchange value: 1 ounce = 1 low-fat meat.

CHICKEN LITTLE

1 broiling or frying chicken, cut in serving pieces	¼ teaspoon dried savory
1 teaspoon salt	¼ teaspoon dried thyme
⅛ teaspoon pepper	1 clove garlic (optional)
½ teaspoon paprika	1 medium onion, sliced
1 tablespoon oil	1 medium green pepper, cut in strips
Juice of one-half lemon	¼ pound mushrooms (optional)
½ cup water	

Sprinkle chicken with salt, pepper, and paprika. Brown in skillet in the oil for 20 minutes, starting with skin side down. Add lemon juice, water, herbs, and garlic. Cover and cook 10 minutes. Add vegetables, cover, and cook 10 minutes longer, or until chicken is tender. Serves 4.

Total recipe contains: 23 grams carbohydrate, 94 grams protein, 47 grams fat, and 891 calories.

One serving (3 ounces of chicken plus ¼ of the vegetables, including mushrooms) contains: 6 grams carbohydrate, 23 grams protein, 12 grams fat, and 223 calories.

Exchange value: 1 serving (3 ounces) = 3 low-fat meat and 1 vegetable.

COMMENT: Remove the bones of the chicken before weighing. A thigh or a drumstick of a 3-pound chicken will usually contain about 1½ ounces of meat.

EAST INDIAN CHICKEN

3 pounds chicken, cut up or quartered	½ teaspoon ground cloves
1 cup low-fat yogurt or buttermilk	½ teaspoon ground cinnamon
1 clove garlic, crushed	1 teaspoon salt
½ teaspoon ground ginger	2 bay leaves

Mix all ingredients and marinate overnight or several hours at least. Remove chicken from yogurt mixture and barbecue over grill or in oven until tender. Serves 4.

One serving (3 ounces) contains: 21 grams protein, 9 grams fat, and 150 calories.

Exchange value: 1 serving (3 ounces) = 1 meat.

COMMENT: It is better to estimate the meat at 1½ ounces per thigh, drumstick, or ½ breast than to remove the bones, which would completely ruin the appearance of the dish.

CHICKEN BREASTS WITH ORANGE SAUCE

1½ pounds chicken breasts, deboned
1 teaspoon salt
½ teaspoon paprika
¼ cup unsaturated margarine

1 cup orange juice
1 tablespoon grated orange rind
1 teaspoon dried tarragon
1 orange, sliced

Sprinkle chicken breasts with salt and paprika; brown lightly in margarine. Add orange juice, rind, and tarragon. Cook in slow oven for 30 minutes. When done, remove chicken and cook sauce over high heat to reduce volume. Serve sauce over chicken and/or steamed rice. Garnish with orange slices. Serves 6.

Total recipe contains: 46 grams carbohydrate, 144 grams protein, and 61 grams fat.

One serving (3 ounces of chicken and ⅙ of total amount of sauce) contains: 8 grams carbohydrate, 24 grams protein, and 10 grams fat.

Exchange value: 3-ounce serving chicken and ⅙ total amount of sauce = 3 low-fat meat and ½ bread.

COMMENT: This dish requires a very simple salad—almost any kind of dressing competes with the piquant flavor of the sauce. Plain lettuce sprinkled with paprika combines better than any.

MINT CHICKEN

3 to 4 pounds chicken, skinned and boned
2 teaspoons salt
¼ teaspoon pepper
1 medium onion, chopped
1 teaspoon oil
1 teaspoon curry powder

2 tablespoons chopped fresh mint or 1 tablespoon dried mint
1 tablespoon thinly sliced fresh ginger root or
1 teaspoon ground ginger
1 tablespoon lime juice

Sprinkle chicken with salt and pepper and set aside. Sauté onions in oil and add curry; stir until onions change color. Add other ingredients, plus ¼ cup water, and simmer until well blended. Add chicken, cover, and simmer about 45 minutes. Serve with rice, using all broth with the rice. Serves 4.

Each serving (3 ounces) contains: 21 grams protein, 9 grams fat, and 150 calories.

Exchange value: 1 serving (3 ounces) = 3 meat.

SMOKED CHICKEN

3 to 4 pounds chicken, skinned
⅓ cup soy sauce
2 tablespoons cooking sherry or 2 tablespoons Chicken Stock (page 73) and ¼ teaspoon vinegar

½ teaspoon smoke flavoring
½ teaspoon grated ginger root or ⅛ teaspoon powdered ginger
1 teaspoon salt
1 tablespoon hoisin sauce

Combine all ingredients in a plastic bag. Marinate for 3 to 4 hours or overnight. Remove chicken from the bag, drain off marinade, and bake chicken at 325° for 1½ hours. Can be served hot or cold. Serves 6.

One ounce of meat contains: 7 grams protein, 3 grams fat, and 50 calories.

Exchange value: 1 ounce = 1 low-fat meat. This marinade is also good when used on turkey or any mild-flavored fowl.

COMMENT: Remove the bones from the portion to be weighed before cooking, or estimate 1½ ounces of meat per drumstick, thigh, or ½ breast.

HANNAH SPIELHOLZ'S CHICKEN

1½ tablespoons oil
3 pounds chicken, deboned
Salt and pepper to taste
2 large cloves garlic, chopped
1 scant teaspoon poultry seasoning

1 teaspoon dried rosemary
1 can (4 ounces) button mushrooms
1 can (4 ounces) black olives
1 can (8 ounces) tomato purée
3 ounces dry sherry

Heat oil in heavy pan and brown chicken on all sides. Sprinkle with salt and pepper. Add garlic, poultry seasoning, and rosemary. Cover and let simmer 10 minutes. Add mushrooms, olives, and tomato purée. Cover and cook over low heat until tomato sauce thickens (about 45 minutes), stirring frequently. Increase heat and add sherry. Cook five minutes more, basting frequently. Serve with rice. Serves 6 to 8.

Total recipe contains: 27 grams carbohydrate, 282 grams protein, 140 grams fat, and 2496 calories.

One serving (⅛ of total) contains: 3 grams carbohydrate, 35 grams protein, 17 grams fat, and 312 calories.

Exchange value: 1 serving (⅛ of total) = 5 low-fat meat exchanges.

NOTE: In this case the carbohydrate content is low and can be disregarded by most patients; however, 17 grams of fat is significant and should be considered in any diet.

OVEN-FRIED CHICKEN

1 frying chicken, about 3 pounds   4 tablespoons cornflake crumbs
Seasoning salt

Skin chicken and sprinkle generously with seasoning salt. Shake in a paper bag with cornflake crumbs. Bake in lightly greased baking pan, uncovered, at 375° for 45 minutes. Leave ample space between pieces and turn once during baking.

One ounce contains: 7 grams protein, 3 grams fat, and 50 calories.
Exchange value: 1 ounce = 1 meat.

COMMENT: Either remove the chicken bones before weighing or estimate at 1½ ounces for one thigh, one drumstick, or a half breast.

CHICKEN WITH PEANUTS

1 cup (150 grams) raw shelled   2 green onions, whole
    peanuts   2 tablespoons cooking sherry
3 quarts boiling water   1 teaspoon sliced ginger root or
1 stewing hen, skinned   ¼ teaspoon powdered ginger
4 teaspoons salt

Soak peanuts in boiling water for 20 to 30 minutes. Place chicken in large covered pan and add all ingredients except peanuts. Simmer 2 hours. Add peanuts with soaking liquid and simmer another 2 hours. Discard onions. Remove any obvious fat. Cut chicken in cubes and serve in bowls with broth. Serves 12.

Total recipe contains: 32 grams carbohydrate, 400 grams protein, 213 grams fat, and 3676 calories.

One serving (1 cup broth, 1 ounce cubed chicken, and 1 ounce, or 2 tablespoons, peanuts) contains: 3 grams carbohydrate, 30 grams protein, 17 grams fat, and 300 calories.

Exchange value: 1 serving = 3 meat and 1 Group A vegetable.

COMMENT: This is an unusual, tasty dish. It is quite filling and can be served with a cottage cheese and fruit salad for a light meal. Raw peanuts are often hard to find and outside the Southeast may seldom be available except in health food stores. The small red Spanish variety is sometimes packaged and sold along with dried beans in other parts of the country.

CHICKEN DIVAN, BRENNAN'S WAY

10 ounces frozen broccoli
Oil
2 pounds cooked chicken, skinned and deboned
1 can (10¾ ounces) condensed cream of chicken soup

¼ cup Mayonnaise (page 68)
½ teaspoon curry powder
½ cup grated Cheddar cheese
6 canned peach halves

Cook the frozen broccoli about half as long as the package directs (it should be bright green and still crisp). Oil the bottom of a glass baking dish (6 × 10) and layer the cooked broccoli over the entire surface. Place the cooked chicken on top. Mix the soup, mayonnaise, and curry until well blended and pour over the chicken. Bake for 10 minutes at 350°. Sprinkle the cheese over the top and return to the oven for another 10 minutes. Put the peaches in a separate dish and warm in the oven for the last 10 minutes. Serve the peach halves as a side dish. This will serve 6 as a main course.

Total recipe contains: 69 grams carbohydrate, 305 grams protein, 169 grams fat, and 3017 calories.

One serving (⅙ of total) contains: 11 grams carbohydrate, 50 grams protein, 28 grams fat, and 496 calories.

Exchange value: 1 serving = 6 meat and 1 Group A vegetable.

SKIP SCHMIDT'S TUMWATER CHICKEN

2 large or 4 small chicken breasts (thighs can be used, but tend to be fat) (about 12 ounces)
½ teaspoon margarine
4 large green onions with top third of green top removed (leeks or other onions may be used)
2 large stalks of celery

8–10 fresh mushrooms
Pinch of garlic or garlic powder to taste
Pepper to taste
Soy sauce to taste (about 3 tablespoons)
Salt to taste (usually not needed because of soy sauce)

Skin and bone chicken. Cut into pieces about 2 inches × 2 inches. Remove any yellow fat. Place ½ teaspoon of margarine in frying pan and, on medium-high heat, brown the chicken slightly. Cover tightly and reduce heat to low. Slice all onion, celery, and mushrooms very thinly. When chicken is done (15 to 25 minutes), remove cover. Place onions, celery, and mushrooms on top of chicken. Add garlic, pepper, and soy sauce to taste (I use about 3 tablespoons of soy) and salt, if necessary. Cover pan tightly. Cook at medium-high heat for about 3 to 5 minutes and serve quickly. Serves 2.

Total recipe contains: 26 grams carbohydrate, 69 grams protein, 11 grams fat, and 480 calories.

One serving (½ of total) contains: 13 grams carbohydrate, 34 grams protein, 6 grams fat, and 240 calories.

Exchange value: 1 serving = 1 vegetable and 2 lean meat.

COMMENT: Combines well with steamed rice. A great low-calorie dinner!

ANGELA'S PHEASANT

1 teaspoon oil
½ pound pheasant, deboned
½ pound fresh mushrooms
1 large green pepper
1 large tomato

⅔ cup steamed rice
2 tablespoons soy sauce
½ teaspoon hoisin sauce
12 pecans, halved

Heat oil very hot in heavy skillet. Dice all ingredients and arrange on platter near stove. Add pheasant to skillet first and stir-fry until brown on all sides. Remove to warm platter. Add mushrooms and stir-fry for

1 to 2 minutes; then add pepper, tomato, and cooked pheasant. Turn off heat.

Place a bed of steamed rice on serving plates. Put pheasant and cooked vegetables on rice, weighing and measuring when necessary. Add soy and hoisin sauces to skillet and heat to simmering. Drizzle over meat and vegetables. Garnish with pecan halves. Serves 2 as a full meal.

Total recipe contains: 50 grams carbohydrate, 70 grams protein, 32 grams fat, and 725 calories.

One serving (½ of total) contains: 25 grams carbohydrate, 33 grams protein, 16 grams fat, and 362 calories.

Exchange value: 1 serving (5 ounces) = 1 meat, 1 Group A vegetable, 1 Group B vegetable, and 9 fat.

Exchange value: 1 serving (½ of total) = 4 low-fat meat, 1 bread, 2 vegetable, and 1 fat.

COMMENT: This is a delicious and quick one-dish meal. Chicken can be substituted for the pheasant but isn't as good.

SWEET AND SOUR PORK

2 pounds pork, cut into bite-size pieces	2 tablespoons soy sauce
	1 tablespoon dry sherry
2 tablespoons soy sauce	Artificial sweetener equivalent to
2 tablespoons flour	1 cup sugar
Oil for deep frying	2 green peppers, cut into strips
2 tablespoons cornstarch	2 tomatoes, cut into wedges
½ cup rice wine vinegar	½ cup pineapple chunks
½ cup water	

Toss the pork with the soy and let sit at least 30 minutes, or preferably overnight. Shake in a bag with the flour and deep-fry until brown and thoroughly cooked. Set aside and keep hot.

Mix cornstarch, vinegar, water, soy sauce, and sherry in a saucepan and boil gently until thickened. Let cool slightly, add sweetener, and mix well. Add green peppers, tomatoes, pineapple, and cooked meat cubes and heat just until the vegetables are warmed through. They should not be cooked. Serve over steamed rice. Serves 6.

Total recipe contains: 73 grams carbohydrate, 173 grams protein, 105 grams fat, 2 grams alcohol.

One serving (⅙ of total) contains: 12 grams carbohydrate, 29 grams protein, 17 grams fat.

Exchange value: 1 serving (⅙ of total) = 3½ medium-fat meats, 1 vegetable, and ½ bread.

SPICED PORK AND VEAL
(from the kitchen of Mrs. Thomas Chinn)

1 pound lean ground pork
½ pound lean ground veal
½ teaspoon pepper
½ teaspoon salt
⅛ teaspoon nutmeg

⅛ teaspoon mace
¼ teaspoon sage
2 tablespoons bread crumbs
2 tablespoons water

Mix all ingredients except water well and shape into patties. Cook in a nonsticking pan until well browned. Add water, cover, and simmer 10 minutes. Serve pan juices along with the meat. The portion for the diabetic can be measured before or after cooking. Serves 6.

Total recipe contains: 8 grams carbohydrate, 134 grams protein, and 63 grams fat.

One serving (⅙ of total) contains: 22 grams protein, 11 grams fat, 185 calories, and negligible carbohydrate.

Exchange value: 1 serving (⅙ of total) = 3 meat.

BARBECUED PORK
(from the kitchen of Mrs. Thomas Chinn)

1 pound lean pork roast (fat trimmed off) or 3 pounds lean ribs
¼ cup soy sauce

2 tablespoons salad oil
⅛ teaspoon cayenne
⅛ teaspoon ground cinnamon
⅛ teaspoon ground cloves

Cut pork into bite-size pieces. Combine ingredients in plastic bag, and marinate 1 to 2 hours. Remove meat from bag and discard marinade. Put meat on small rack or skewers and bake at 325° for 1 hour. Serves 4.

Total recipe contains: 6 grams carbohydrate, 87 grams protein, and 74 grams fat.

One serving (3 ounces) contains: 21 grams protein, 15 grams fat, and 225 calories.

Exchange value: 1 serving (3 ounces) = 2 meat.

KATIE'S PERSIAN LAMB
(from the kitchen of Mrs. Thomas Ghavamian)

2 medium eggplants
1 teaspoon salt
2 tablespoons oil
1½ pounds lamb (cut from leg into stew-meat pieces, all fat removed), cut in 1-inch cubes
1 medium white onion, finely chopped
½ teaspoon cinnamon
½ teaspoon pepper
¼ teaspoon nutmeg
3 dashes paprika
1 can (6 ounces) tomato paste
2 cups water
4 tablespoons lemon juice
6 tablespoons margarine
2 medium tomatoes, cut into wedges

Cut unpeeled eggplants into 1-inch slices, lengthwise. Wash, and sprinkle with salt, and let stand 20 minutes to take out bitterness.

Add oil to 4-quart saucepan or large skillet. Add meat, onion, and seasonings and sauté. Then add tomato paste, water, and lemon juice to meat and simmer over low heat for about 45 minutes to an hour, or until meat is tender. Wash salt off eggplant and dry. Add margarine to another skillet and sauté eggplant separately until browned and tender. About 15 minutes before meat is done, add eggplant and tomato wedges to meat sauce and let cook very slowly (simmer) for these last 15 minutes. Serve with steamed rice or noodles. Serves 6.

Total recipe contains: 88 grams carbohydrate, 153 grams protein, 135 grams fat, and 2220 calories.

One serving (⅙ total) contains: 15 grams carbohydrate, 26 grams protein, 23 grams fat, and 370 calories.

Exchange value: 1 serving = 2 Group B vegetables and 4 meat.

COMMENT: Chicken may be substituted for the lamb.

EPICUREAN LAMB
(from the kitchen of Hannah W. Spielholz)

½ cup chopped onions
1 tablespoon corn oil
1 can (4 ounces) sliced mushrooms
2½ cups (500 grams) cooked lamb, cut in chunks
1 cup cooked rice (⅓ cup uncooked)
1 can (2½ cups) tomatoes
1 teaspoon salt
⅛ teaspoon pepper
½ teaspoon curry powder
¼ cup Parmesan cheese

Cook onion in oil until golden. Add drained mushrooms and brown lightly. Combine all ingredients except cheese and place in greased 1½-quart casserole. Sprinkle with cheese and bake at 400° for 45 minutes, covered; uncover and bake 10 minutes. Serves 6.

Total recipe contains: 65 grams carbohydrate, 169 grams protein, and 63 grams fat.

One serving (⅙ of total) contains: 11 grams carbohydrate, 28 grams protein, 11 grams fat, and 255 calories.

Exchange value: 1 serving (⅙ of total) = 4 meat, ½ bread, and 1 Group A vegetable.

LAMB AND SPRING ONIONS

1½ pounds lean lamb, thinly sliced
¾ teaspoon Chinese Five Spice
1 egg white
2 cloves garlic, mashed
6 slices fresh ginger

2 tablespoons soy sauce
6 tablespoons sherry
2 tablespoons water
10 green onions
2 tablespoons corn oil

Marinate lamb in Five Spice, egg white, garlic, ginger, and soy sauce for 20 to 30 minutes using a plastic bag. Heat oil in heavy skillet until very hot; add lamb and stir until meat browns. Remove lamb and keep warm. Add marinade, sherry, water, and whole onions to skillet. Stir and simmer 3 to 5 minutes. Add meat and serve. Serves 6.

Total recipe contains: 30 grams carbohydrate, 140 grams protein, 63 grams fat, and 1260 calories.

One serving (⅙ of total) contains: 5 grams carbohydrate, 23 grams protein, 11 grams fat, and 210 calories.

Exchange value: 1 serving = 3 meat and 1 Group A vegetable.

COMMENT: If necessary, ⅛ teaspoon powdered cinnamon, ⅛ teaspoon powdered cloves, and ¼ teaspoon anise seed can be used instead of Chinese Five Spice. The effect is not quite the same, but it is acceptable.

GROUND BEEF WITH BUTTER BEANS
(from the kitchen of Mrs. Dorothy Rockwell)

1 pound lean ground beef	1 can (15 ounces) butter beans
1 medium onion, sliced	(large limas)
1 green pepper, cut in strips	Salt and pepper to taste

Brown ground beef. Add onion and green pepper. Cook only until onion and pepper are cooked but still crisp. Add butter beans with liquid, and heat. Add salt and pepper to taste. Serves 4.

Total recipe contains: 68 grams carbohydrate, 114 grams protein, 46 grams fat, and 1160 calories.

One serving (¼ of total) contains: 17 grams carbohydrate, 28 grams protein, 12 grams fat, and 290 calories.

Exchange value: 1 serving (¼ of total) = 1 bread and 4 meat.

BEEF SPINACH SCRAMBLE

2 pounds very lean ground beef	¼ teaspoon oregano
2 tablespoons corn oil	½ teaspoon salt
1 medium onion, chopped	1 bunch (½ pound) spinach,
1 clove garlic, mashed	chopped
1¼ teaspoons nutmeg	4 eggs
¼ teaspoon pepper	

Brown ground beef in oil. Add onions and garlic. Cook over low heat until onion is clear. Add seasoning and mix well. Stir in spinach. Cook over very low heat for 3 to 5 minutes. Add eggs and stir. Heat until eggs set. Serves about 6.

Total recipe contains: 16 grams carbohydrate, 225 grams protein, and 144 grams fat.

One serving (⅙ of total) contains: 3 grams carbohydrate, 37 grams protein, 24 grams fat, and 375 calories.

Exchange value: 1 serving (⅙ of total) = 5 meat and 1 Group A vegetable.

GINGER BEEF WITH LITTLE GREEN ONIONS

1½ pounds lean beef, thinly sliced	12 small green onions
2 tablespoons soy sauce	2 tablespoons corn oil
1 clove garlic, mashed	3 tablespoons cooking sherry
8 slices fresh ginger root	3 tablespoons water

Marinate beef in 1 tablespoon of the soy sauce, garlic, and ginger for 30 minutes. Chop green onions into 1-inch pieces. Heat oil in a heavy pan and add onions. Cook until limp. Remove onion. Add beef mixture and cook until beef browns lightly. Add sherry, water, and remaining soy sauce. Return onions to pan and heat to serving temperature. Serves 4.

Total recipe contains: 29 grams carbohydrate, 149 grams protein, 60 grams fat, and 1240 calories.

One serving (¼ of total) contains: 7 grams carbohydrate, 37 grams protein, 15 grams fat, and 310 calories.

Exchange value: 1 serving (¼ of total) = 5 meat and 1 Group B vegetable.

BEEF WITH BROCCOLI
(from the kitchen of Mrs. Thomas Chinn)

1 pound broccoli	½ pound lean beef
1 tablespoon cornstarch	1 tablespoon corn oil
2 tablespoons soy sauce	½ teaspoon salt
1 tablespoon sesame oil	2 tablespoons water
1 tablespoon sherry	

Cut broccoli spears and then slit into two to four sections. Slice stalk into thin slices. Mix cornstarch, soy sauce, sesame oil, sherry, and beef. Heat ½ tablespoon of the corn oil in frying pan until hot. Stir-fry broccoli and salt for 1 minute. Add 2 tablespoons water and cook for 2 minutes more; remove from heat and set aside. Again, heat ½ tablespoon corn oil in frying pan until hot. Stir-fry beef mixture for 2 minutes. Add broccoli to beef mixture and stir well for 2 minutes. Serve hot. Serves 3.

Total recipe contains: 27 grams carbohydrate, 59 grams protein, 38 grams fat, and 690 calories.

One serving (⅓ of total) contains: 9 grams carbohydrate, 20 grams protein, 13 grams fat, and 230 calories.

(continued)

Exchange value: 1 serving (⅓ of total) = 3 meat and 1 Group B vegetable.

COMMENT: Fresh asparagus can be substituted for broccoli. Calculations remain the same.

BEEF WINE STEW
(from the kitchen of Hannah W. Spielholz)

2 pounds lean stewing beef, cubed
1 tablespoon corn oil
Salt and pepper
2 cloves garlic

Large pinch of thyme
1 cup tomato purée
½ cup dry red wine
2 onions, thinly sliced
2 large carrots, thinly sliced

Brown beef thoroughly in corn oil in heavy pan. Season well with salt and pepper (approximately 1 teaspoon salt and ¼ teaspoon pepper). Add chopped garlic, thyme, tomato purée, and wine; cover and simmer for 1 hour, or 15 minutes in pressure cooker. (If cooked under pressure, reduce heat rapidly under cold running water.) Add onions and carrots and simmer gently until tender (45 minutes). Adjust seasonings. Serve with rice. Serves 6.

Total recipe contains: 62 grams carbohydrate, 202 grams protein, 31 grams fat, and 1800 calories.

One serving (⅙ of total) contains: 10 grams carbohydrate, 34 grams protein, 14 grams fat, and 300 calories.

Exchange value: 1 serving (⅙ of total) = 5 meat and 1 Group B vegetable.

TOMATO MEAT LOAF
(from the kitchen of Mrs. Dorothy Rockwell)

1 can (7½ ounces) tomato sauce, unsweetened
2 pounds ground meat
⅓ cup saltines (8 crushed)
¾ cup onion, chopped
½ cup fresh parsley, chopped (or ¼ cup dried)

1 egg
1 tablespoon Worcestershire sauce
½ teaspoon dry mustard
½ teaspoon salt
¼ teaspoon pepper

Combine ¾ cup tomato sauce with other ingredients. Meat loaf should be baked in a broiler pan so fat can drain off. Cover with aluminum foil tent so it will retain moisture. Bake in a 375° oven approximately 1¼ hours. During last 5 minutes remove aluminum foil and spoon remaining tomato sauce over meat loaf. Do not overcook or meat will be dry. Serves 8.

Total recipe contains: 59 grams carbohydrate, 181 grams protein, 105 grams fat, and 1810 calories.

Each serving (⅛ of total) contains: 7 grams carbohydrate, 23 grams protein, 13 grams fat, and 235 calories.

Exchange value: 1 serving (⅛ of total) = ½ bread and 3 meat.

COMMENT: To approximate eight equal servings, mound meat loaf in a half-moon shape and cut into eight equal pie-shaped pieces.

ROASTED SOYBEANS

1 cup dry soybeans	½ cup soy sauce
2 quarts water	2 tablespoons molasses
1 can (3 ounces) bamboo shoots	¼ teaspoon aniseeds

Place beans and 2 cups of the water in a pan and freeze. When ready to cook remove from freezer and add remaining water. Heat to boiling. Reduce heat and simmer about 1 hour or until tender. Beans can be cooked without prior freezing, but it takes much longer. Add more water as necessary. When beans are tender, add other ingredients and bake at 350° for 1 hour. Beans should be coated with sauce, but no liquid should remain in the pan. Serves 6.

Total recipe contains: 100 grams carbohydrate, 70 grams protein, 35 grams fat, and 1020 calories.

One serving (⅙ of total) contains: 17 grams carbohydrate, 12 grams protein, 6 grams fat, and 170 calories.

Exchange value: 1 serving (⅙ of total) = 1 bread and 2 meat.

COMMENT: Soybeans make a satisfactory meat substitute. Although they are relatively high in carbohydrate, this is tempered by the amount of protein and fat they also contain. The fat is, of course, mostly unsaturated.

Eggs

Some of the following recipes utilize only the whites of eggs in order to eliminate the saturated fat contained in egg yolks. If you are permitted saturated fat, whole eggs can be used in any of the recipes and the yellow coloring omitted. Remember that 5 grams of fat, 3 grams of protein, and 60 calories are present in an average egg yolk, and these amounts must be added for each egg yolk added. Numerous nutrients are added as well. Egg substitutes can be used if desired.

EGGS WITH SCALLOPS

1 pound scallops
3 tablespoons finely chopped leek
2 tablespoons cooking oil

6 egg whites
¼ teaspoon yellow food coloring

Add scallops and leek to cooking oil. Sauté gently for 5 to 6 minutes or until the scallops are done. Beat egg whites and add yellow food coloring; pour over scallops. Stir until eggs are done as you like. Serve immediately. Makes 4 generous servings.

Total recipe contains: 20 grams carbohydrate, 90 grams protein, 30 grams fat, and 680 calories.

One serving (¼ of total) contains: 5 grams carbohydrate, 22 grams protein, 7 grams fat, and 170 calories.

Exchange value: 1 serving (¼ of total) = 3 meat and 1 Group A vegetable.

COMMENT: Shrimp may be substituted for the scallops. This dish is good for breakfast or brunch, or can be served with toasted English muffins, a green salad, and a vegetable for a full meal.

EGG FLOWER SOUP

4 egg whites
¼ teaspoon yellow food coloring
6 cups Chicken Stock (page 73)

2½ teaspoons salt
½ teaspoon sugar
¼ cup sliced mushrooms

Beat egg whites with food coloring until well mixed but not too frothy. Bring broth, salt, and sugar to boiling and add mushrooms. While broth is simmering, pour in egg mixture in a fine stream, stirring constantly. Remove from heat and serve immediately. Makes about 6 cups.

Total recipe contains: 6 grams carbohydrate, 38 grams protein, 0 grams fat, and 150 calories.

One cup (⅙ of total) contains: 6 grams protein, 25 calories, and negligible fat and carbohydrate.

Exchange value: 1 cup (⅙ of total) = 1 meat.

QUICHE LORRAINE

¼ pound mushrooms	1½ cups evaporated skim milk
1 tablespoon margarine	6 ounces Swiss cheese, thinly
¼ teaspoon yellow food coloring	sliced
6 egg whites, lightly beaten	Nutmeg

Combine all ingredients except nutmeg and pour into glass baking dish. Sprinkle top with nutmeg and bake in slow oven (325°) for 20 to 30 minutes or until consistency of custard. A toothpick can be inserted near the edge to test for doneness; if it comes out clean, the center will be the right consistency. Serves 6 adequately as a main course. The quiche can be served with a green salad and low-calorie dressing.

Total recipe contains: 46 grams carbohydrate, 97 grams protein, 61 grams fat, and 1116 calories.

One serving (⅙ of total) contains: 8 grams carbohydrate, 16 grams protein, 10 grams fat, and 186 calories.

Exchange value: 1 serving (⅙ of total) = 2 meat and ½ bread.

COMMENT: I have altered the classic quiche recipe to decrease the amount of saturated fat and increase the unsaturated fat. It still contains some saturated fat, but the ratio of unsaturated to saturated is acceptable.

SCRAMBLED EGGS

1 tablespoon cooking oil or
  margarine
2 egg whites
4 to 5 drops yellow food coloring

2 tablespoons evaporated skim
  milk
⅛ teaspoon salt

Heat oil in small pan. Beat remaining ingredients and add to hot oil. Stir briskly until properly set. Serves 1.

Total recipe contains: 3 grams carbohydrate, 9 grams protein, 14 grams fat, and 174 calories.

Exchange value: 1 serving (total recipe) = 1 meat and 2 fat.

For low-fat diets, omit oil and cook in top of double boiler. This variation contains: 3 grams carbohydrate, 9 grams protein, and 50 calories.

Exchange value: 1 low-fat meat.

If whole eggs are used, the product contains: 3 grams carbohydrate, 12 grams protein, 24 grams fat, and 275 calories.

Exchange value: 2 medium-fat meat and 3 fat.

FANCY SCRAMBLED EGGS

2 tablespoons unsaturated
  margarine
2 tablespoons sesame seeds
6 whole eggs

1 tablespoon Bourbon
4 tablespoons evaporated skim
  milk
1 tablespoon soy sauce

Gently heat margarine in heavy skillet and add sesame seeds. Toast lightly. Beat eggs, bourbon, and milk. Add to sesame seeds and stir until properly set. Garnish each serving with 1 teaspoon soy sauce. Serves three or four.

Total recipe contains: 13 grams carbohydrate, 50 grams protein, and 69 grams fat.

One serving (¼ of total) contains: 3 grams carbohydrate, 12 grams protein, 17 grams fat, and 210 calories.

Exchange value: 1 serving (¼ of total) = 2 meat and 1 fat.

For low-fat diets, reduce margarine to 1 tablespoon and sesame seeds to 1 tablespoon. Omit egg yolks and include ¼ teaspoon yellow food coloring. In this case entire dish contains: 12 grams carbohydrate, 26 grams protein, and 16 grams fat.

One serving (¼ of total) contains: 3 grams carbohydrate, 7 grams protein, and 4 grams fat.

Exchange value: 1 serving (¼ of total) = 1 medium-fat meat.

CHAPTER 9

Vegetables

- Cooked Greens
- Bok Choy
- Mom's Turnip Greens
- Broccoli and Mushrooms
- Dilled Cabbage and Beans
- Sesame Chard
- Mushrooms and Peapods
- Eggplant and Tomato
- Mushrooms and Asparagus
- Gingered Carrots
- Red and White

- Squash and Mushrooms
- Green Peppers
- Baked Red Peppers
- Baked Potato
- Broiled Eggplant
- Mom's Eggplant
- Mixed Squash
- Evelyn's Spinach Pie
- Green Celery
- Zucchini

It is ironic that the Group A, or low-carbohydrate, vegetables are among the least often enjoyed by many families. An especially large portion of this chapter is devoted to recipes for preparing these vegetables. Many of them are excellent sources of vitamins and minerals and should be used daily in diets for the whole family as well as the diabetic member.

LEAFY GREEN VEGETABLES

Outside the Southeast, greens are rarely eaten except in salads. This is unfortunate, as many of them are quite tasty and all are excellent sources of vitamin A and the B complex.

The following basic recipe is suitable for cooking most greens. The most common error is to overcook. When this occurs, the color changes from a bright green to a yellowish green and the flavor becomes much stronger and somewhat altered. If you've never eaten a cooked green vegetable except canned or frozen spinach, you have a pleasant surprise in store. If the greens are young and tender, which they rarely are unless you either grow your own or shop in an Oriental market area, they will cook completely in less than 3 minutes. If they are tough, cooking will take somewhat longer, but never longer than 10 minutes.

Because of the very low calorie content of greens, it is possible to use larger amounts of fat and other seasoning sauces than is practical with many other vegetables. In these recipes the fat content has been kept as low as possible without altering the flavor of the finished dish unnecessarily. If your diet permits additional fat, by all means use it, but remember to increase the calories accordingly. If your diet requires the use of extra unsaturated fat, most of the cooked vegetables here—especially the greens and squashes—make an ideal vehicle. To avoid altered flavor, add oil immediately before serving. Remember that 1 teaspoon of fat carries 45 calories and 5 grams of fat and is equal to one fat exchange.

COOKED GREENS

Wash, but do not shake, one bunch of greens for each two members of your family. Heat a heavy pan and add 1 teaspoon cooking oil or bacon drippings for each bunch of greens. Add the greens and cook quickly, stirring every minute or so. Salt to taste and set off heat when they are well wilted but not overdone. Let sit in covered pan for 5 to 10 minutes. They will continue to cook a bit after you've removed them from the heat. Serve with corn bread and fish or pork.

If fat intake is very limited, count one-half fat exchange, or 2.5 grams, for each serving. Each serving contains about 35 calories.

BOK CHOY
(Chinese cabbage)

2 cups Chicken Stock (page 73) or   ⅛ teaspoon pepper
   canned chicken broth   1½ teaspoon salt
1 small onion, diced   2 cups bok choy, diagonally sliced

Heat stock and seasonings to boiling; add bok choy, cover pot, and turn off heat. Remove cover occasionally to test. The bok should be crisp but tender. Serve with French dressing or plain. The broth can be served separately as clear soup.

One cup of broth or ½ cup of vegetable contains vitamins A and B and trace minerals, but negligible carbohydrate, protein, and fat. Consider only the dressing used.

COMMENT: This makes a good filler dish to combine with meats and other high-calorie entrees and also combines well with Italian-style casseroles such as lasagne, because it permits more calories, carbohydrate, and fat to be taken in the main dish.

MOM'S TURNIP GREENS

Cut 2 bunches turnips with roots into quarters and simmer in ¼ cup water and ½ teaspoon salt. Wash greens and remove tough stems while roots are cooking. About 5 minutes before serving time, add greens and continue simmering for 5 minutes. Add extra salt, if necessary, and 1 teaspoon bacon drippings or other fat before serving. Garnish with black pepper. Serves 4.

Greens contain: iron, vitamins A and B, negligible carbohydrate, negligible protein, and negligible fat.

One serving (½ cup) of roots: 7 grams carbohydrate, 2 grams protein, 0 grams fat, and 35 calories.

Exchange value: 1 serving (½ cup) roots = 1 group B vegetable.

Stir-Fried Mixed Vegetables

When families are confronted with strange vegetables for the first time, it usually requires some salesmanship even to get the dish tasted, let alone eaten. The Chinese custom of blending several vegetables in one dish often lets a new vegetable pass almost unnoticed. If you're trying a new vegetable, make up the remainder of the dish from familiar things. The family is less likely to balk this way.

Stir-frying involves using a heavy pan with a small amount of fat. Vegetables are added according to length of cooking time required and stirred constantly while they fry in the hot pan. The vegetables are seared and caramelized by the high heat, adding a pleasantly different flavor.

Mixtures are limited only by your imagination and the caloric restrictions in your diet. Several recipes are included below as examples. If it's an especially hectic day, leftover meat, fowl, or fish can be added at the last minute for a one-dish meal. If the fat content of your diet is limited, try this method of cooking either fresh or frozen vegetables.

The dishes appear more interesting if the colors are mixed and if the vegetables are sliced diagonally.

BROCCOLI AND MUSHROOMS

1 teaspoon oil
2 cups diagonally sliced celery
2 cups diagonally sliced broccoli
2 cups (about ½ pound) diagonally sliced mushrooms
1 large green pepper

⅛ teaspoon garlic powder
⅛ teaspoon curry powder
½ teaspoon salt
1 tablespoon lemon juice or cider vinegar

Heat pan; add oil, then celery, broccoli, mushrooms, and pepper. Stir-fry 3 to 4 minutes. Add seasonings and lemon juice or cider vinegar and turn off heat. Let stand 3 to 4 minutes longer. Serves 4 to 6 generously.

Total recipe contains: 26 grams carbohydrate, 14 grams protein, 5 grams fat, and 245 calories.

One serving (½ cup) contains: 4 grams carbohydrate, 2 grams protein, 1 gram fat, and 35 calories.

Exchange value: 1 serving (½ cup) = 1 Group A vegetable.

DILLED CABBAGE AND BEANS

1 teaspoon oil
8 cups shredded cabbage
1½ cups French green beans

½ teaspoon dried dill weed
¼ teaspoon salt

Heat oil in heavy pan; add remaining ingredients and stir quickly until cabbage is slightly wilted. Cover and steam for 5 more minutes. Add additional water (not more than 2 or 3 tablespoons) if vegetables appear dry. Serves 6.

Total recipe contains: 49 grams carbohydrate, 13 grams protein, 5 grams fat, 250 calories, and vitamins A, B, and C.

One serving (1 cup) contains: 8 grams carbohydrate, 2 grams protein, 1 gram fat, and 50 calories.

Exchange value: 1 serving (1 cup) = 1 Group B vegetable.

SESAME CHARD

Wash about 1 pound Swiss chard and remove stems. Chop into bite-size pieces. Heat a large, heavy pan moderately hot and add 1 teaspoon margarine. Stir-fry chard about 2 minutes or just until well wilted. Season with salt and garnish heavily with toasted sesame seeds. Serves 4.

Total recipe (2 cups) contains: 16 grams carbohydrate, 8 grams protein, 4 grams fat, and 140 calories.

One serving (½ cup) contains: 4 grams carbohydrate, 2 grams protein, 1 gram fat, and 35 calories.

Exchange value: 1 serving (½ cup) = 1 Group A vegetable. This is a good source of vitamins A and B and iron.

MUSHROOMS AND PEAPODS

1 teaspoon cooking oil	½ pound fresh mushrooms,
½ pound edible peapods with	diagonally sliced
stems removed (or 10-ounce	1 tablespoon soy sauce
package frozen)	1 teaspoon grated fresh ginger or
1 cup diagonally sliced celery	¼ teaspoon powdered ginger

Heat heavy pan very hot and add oil. Add peapods first (if frozen, allow to cook until thawed before adding next vegetable), then celery, and finally mushrooms (if canned mushrooms are used, add when cooking is completed and allow only to heat through). Stir-fry about 2 minutes after mushrooms are added. Lower heat to lowest setting and add soy sauce and ginger. Let simmer 2 to 3 minutes longer. Serve at once. Serves 6.

Total recipe contains: 37 grams carbohydrate, 14 grams protein, 5 grams fat, and 275 calories.

One serving (½ cup) contains: 7 grams carbohydrate, 2 grams protein, 1 gram fat, and 45 calories.

Exchange value: 1 serving (½ cup) = 1 Group B vegetable.

EGGPLANT AND TOMATO

1 tablespoon cooking oil
1 eggplant, unpeeled and diced
1 small onion, chopped
½ teaspoon salt
Dash of pepper

½ teaspoon dried basil
2 large tomatoes, peeled and
   diced
Parmesan cheese

Put oil in heavy frying pan with cover; add eggplant and onion and sauté 4 to 5 minutes. Add salt, pepper, and basil; cook covered 10 minutes. Add tomatoes and cook uncovered 5 minutes, stirring occasionally. Raise heat during last minute of cooking to evaporate excess moisture. Sprinkle with Parmesan cheese. Serves 4.

Total recipe contains: 37 grams carbohydrate, 9 grams protein, 15 grams fat, and 320 calories.

One serving (½ cup) contains: 9 grams carbohydrate, 2 grams protein, 4 grams fat, and 80 calories.

Exchange value: 1 serving (½ cup) = 1 Group B vegetable and 1 fat.

MUSHROOMS AND ASPARAGUS

1 teaspoon oil
2 cups diagonally sliced
   asparagus

½ pound fresh mushrooms,
   diagonally sliced
Salt and pepper

Heat pan; add 1 teaspoon oil, then add asparagus. Stir-fry 1 to 2 minutes; add mushrooms and continue to stir for 2 more minutes. Add salt and pepper to taste. Serves 4.

Total recipe contains: 17 grams carbohydrate, 13 grams protein, 5 grams fat, and 140 calories.

One serving (½ cup) contains: 4 grams carbohydrate, 3 grams protein, 1 gram fat, and 35 calories.

Exchange value: 1 serving (½ cup) = 1 Group A vegetable.

GINGERED CARROTS

1 teaspoon oil
4 cups carrots diagonally sliced ⅛
   inch thick
1 tablespoon (10 grams)
   crystallized ginger

2 tablespoons wine vinegar
¼ teaspoon salt
⅛ teaspoon garlic powder
2 tablespoons parsley, chopped

Heat oil in heavy pan and add carrots. Stir-fry for 1 to 2 minutes. Add remaining ingredients; cover and cook over low heat for about 15 minutes or until carrots are tender. Serves 6.

Total recipe contains: 52 grams carbohydrate, 6 grams protein, 5 grams fat, and 300 calories.

One serving (½ cup) contains: 9 grams carbohydrate, 1 gram protein, 1 gram fat, and 50 calories.

This recipe also contains a large amount of vitamin A.

Exchange value: 1 serving (½ cup) = 1 Group B vegetable.

RED AND WHITE

1 teaspoon oil
1½ cups diagonally sliced celery
2 cups diagonally sliced cauliflower buds and leaves (½ inch thick)

1 large red bell pepper, diced (about ½ cup)
Dash liquid hot pepper
½ teaspoon salt

Heat pan and add oil. Add celery, then cauliflower, and then pepper. Stir-fry for 3 to 4 minutes. Add seasonings and remove from heat. Let stand covered another 3 to 4 minutes. All vegetables should remain crisp. Serves 4.

Total recipe contains: 16 grams carbohydrate, 7 grams protein, 5 grams fat, and 140 calories.

One serving (½ cup) contains: 4 grams carbohydrate, 2 grams protein, 1 gram fat, and 35 calories.

Exchange value: 1 serving (½ cup) = 1 Group A vegetable.

SQUASH AND MUSHROOMS

1 tablespoon unsaturated margarine
1 pound summer squash
¼ pound mushrooms
1 small onion, finely chopped

Dash black pepper (more if desired)
½ teaspoon salt
¼ teaspoon dried dill weed
¼ cup green pepper, chopped

Heat margarine in heavy skillet until hot; add sliced squash, mushrooms, and onion and sauté 2 to 3 minutes, uncovered. Add seasonings, cover, and cook for 5 to 6 minutes, keeping the heat rather high. Add green pepper and serve. Serves 6.

Total recipe contains: 27 grams carbohydrate, 9 grams protein, 11 grams fat, 240 calories and vitamins A, B, and C.

One serving (⅙ of total) contains: 4 grams carbohydrate, 2 grams protein, 2 grams fat, and 40 calories.

Exchange value: 1 serving = 1 Group A vegetable and ½ fat.

Miscellaneous Vegetables

GREEN PEPPERS

1 tablespoon unsaturated margarine

4 bell peppers, cut in quarters, seeds and white membrane removed

1 clove garlic

1½ teaspoons salt

⅛ teaspoon pepper

1 teaspoon dried oregano

Heat margarine in heavy skillet and add peppers and garlic; sauté 2 to 3 minutes. Sprinkle with seasoning; cover and simmer 10 minutes. Discard garlic. Serves 4 as a side dish.

Total recipe contains: 14 grams carbohydrate, 5 grams protein, 11 grams fat, and 200 calories.

One serving (4 pieces) contains: 4 grams carbohydrate, 1 gram protein, 3 grams fat, 50 calories, and vitamins A and C.

Exchange value: 1 serving (4 pieces) = 1 Group A vegetable.

BAKED RED PEPPERS

3 cans (7½ ounces each) red pimientos

½ cup Medego Villari (page 43)

Oil the bottom of a glass serving dish. Layer with drained pimientos. Sprinkle with about ¼ of the medego mix. Continue until all ingredients have been layered. Bake at 350° for 20 minutes. Garnish the top with a little chopped parsley or chives before serving. Serves 8.

Total recipe contains: 53 grams carbohydrate, 16 grams protein, 12 grams fat, and 345 calories.

One serving (⅛ of total) contains: 7 grams carbohydrate, 2 grams protein, 2 grams fat, and 42 calories.

Exchange value: 1 serving (⅛ of total) = 1 vegetable and ½ fat.

COMMENT: Good hot or cold. It makes a pretty table with spinach.

BAKED POTATO

1 medium potato (100 grams) per serving
½ cup dry cottage cheese
¼ cup vegetable oil

¼ cup evaporated skim milk
2 tablespoons chopped chives, for garnish

Bake potato in usual manner. As soon as it is done, split lengthwise and scoop out about a quarter or more of the potato and discard. (Those on weighed diets should weigh the potato after this has been removed and adjust calculations accordingly.) Put cottage cheese, oil, and milk in a blender and blend until smooth (or pass through a food mill if you have no blender). Use to replace discarded potato. Garnish with chives.

One potato (100 grams) contains: 17 grams carbohydrate, 2 grams protein, and 76 calories.

One tablespoon cheese mixture: 4 grams fat and 35 calories. The carbohydrate and protein content of the cheese mixture can be disregarded, provided not more than 2 tablespoons are used.

Exchange value: 1 bread and 1 fat.

COMMENT: When high-carbohydrate foods such as potato are served, an effort should be made to replace some of the starch with protein and/or fat. This permits the allowed carbohydrate to be taken in a more nutritious form, such as whole-grain bread or cereals.

BROILED EGGPLANT

Cut a large eggplant crosswise into slices about ¾ inch thick. Brush each side with margarine and sprinkle with salt, pepper, and paprika. Broil 6 to 8 minutes on each side.

Two slices contain: 5 grams carbohydrate, 1 gram protein, 3 grams fat, and 50 calories.

Exchange value: 2 slices = 1 Group A vegetable and ½ fat.

MOM'S EGGPLANT
(from the kitchen of Mrs. L. W. Middleton)

1 large eggplant
2 tablespoons flour
1 teaspoon pork sausage
  seasoning with sage

1 teaspoon oil
Salt and pepper, if necessary

Peel and slice eggplant. Simmer until tender in ¼ cup water in covered pan. Add flour and seasoning and stir until smooth. Add extra salt and pepper if necessary; the mixture should be quite spicy with a distinct flavor of sage. Heat well-seasoned cast-iron or other heavy griddle to about pancake-cooking temperature. Drop mixture by spoonfuls onto oiled griddle and brown like pancakes. Serves 4.

Total recipe contains: 27 grams carbohydrate, 6 grams protein, and 5 grams fat.

One serving (¼ of total) contains: 7 grams carbohydrate, 1 gram protein, 1 gram fat, and 40 calories.

Exchange value: 1 serving (¼ of total) = 1 Group B vegetable.

MIXED SQUASH

3 small zucchini
3 small crookneck squash
¼ cup boiling salted water
1 tablespoon salad oil

2 tablespoons lemon juice
½ teaspoon dried oregano
Salt and pepper

Slice squash lengthwise and cook in the salted water for about 8 minutes. Drain. Blend remaining ingredients and pour over hot squash. Let marinate about 5 minutes. Squash can then be lifted from dressing. Serves 6.

Total recipe contains: 24 grams carbohydrate, 6 grams protein, 14 grams fat, and 120 calories.

One serving (⅙ of total) contains: 4 grams carbohydrate, 1 gram protein, 2 grams fat, and 20 calories.

Exchange value: 1 serving = 1 Group A vegetable.

If dressing is eaten, count 45 calories per tablespoon and 5 grams of fat (or 1 fat exchange).

EVELYN'S SPINACH PIE

1 small onion, finely chopped
1 tablespoon olive oil
2 packages (10 ounces each)
  frozen, chopped spinach
  (thawed and drained)
½ cup chopped ripe olives

1 large clove garlic, grated
Salt and pepper to taste
½ cup Medego Villari (page 43)
½ cup chopped pimiento,
  preferably fresh

Sauté the onion in the olive oil until clear. Increase heat to high and add spinach. Stir-fry the spinach until it is free of all excess moisture. Remove from heat and add the olives, garlic, salt, and pepper. Mix well and pour into a deep 10-inch glass pie dish. Arrange the medego around the edge as a crust. Layer the chopped pimiento just inside this ring, leaving a circle of the green spinach showing in the center. A very pretty dish. Bake 20 minutes at 350°. Serves 8.

Total recipe contains: 56 grams carbohydrate, 31 grams protein, 32 grams fat, and 560 calories.

One serving (⅛ of total) contains: 7 grams carbohydrate, 4 grams protein, 4 grams fat, and 70 calories.

Exchange value: 1 serving (⅛ of total) = 1 Group A vegetable and 1 fat.

NOTE: Jess Spielholz describes this as "the most civilized way spinach can be served."

GREEN CELERY

½ cup milk
½ teaspoon salt
2 cups diagonally sliced celery,
  outside stalks

Celery leaves, chopped
Paprika for garnish

Cook milk, salt, and celery stalks in top of double boiler for 5 minutes. Add chopped celery leaves and cook 3 minutes longer. Garnish with paprika. Serves 4.

One serving (½ cup) contains: 30 calories.

Exchange value: 1 serving (½ cup) = 1 Group A vegetable.

ZUCCHINI

1 ½ cups chopped celery
1 cup chopped onion
1 tablespoon unsaturated
  margarine

¼ cup Chicken Stock (page 73)
3 cups sliced zucchini
¼ cup cooking sherry
Salt to taste

Sauté celery and onion in margarine; add stock and zucchini. Simmer for barely 5 minutes. Zucchini should still be crisp. Add sherry and salt before serving. Makes about 5 cups.

Total recipe contains: 33 grams carbohydrate, 7 grams protein, 11 grams fat, and 250 calories.

One serving (½ cup) contains: 3 grams carbohydrate, 1 gram protein, 1 gram fat, and 25 calories.

Exchange value: 1 serving (½ cup) = 1 Group A vegetable.

COMMENT: This dish is considerably more flavorful with additional fat, and if your diet permits, by all means increase the fat, but don't forget to increase also the amount of calories and fat in your calculations.

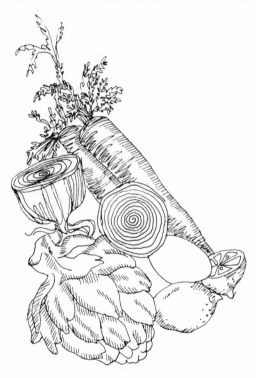

CHAPTER 10

Breads

Fresh, hot bread was a part of every meal of my childhood, and I still consider it an essential part of any really elegant meal. Fresh bread begins to add an extra dimension to a meal as soon as the aroma leaves the oven. Most of the breads included here have been made in my kitchen with such regularity that a measuring spoon or cup is totally unnecessary.

One of the boring chores in writing these recipes for publication was the transformation of my "dump and stir" method of baking bread into precise measure. My young friend Sarah Reade has leaned over my kitchen counter many hours as I carelessly threw together a little of this and a little of that for the bread of the day. This lack of precision has led her to say, "Is that going to turn out?" on more than one occasion. To my delight, she now uses this method in her own kitchen and the dishes "turn out" with impressive regularity. So I encourage the art of estimation. Learn what a half teaspoon of salt looks like, how much liquid is a cupful, and so forth. You will cook much more often and much more creatively.

There are dishes that I don't fool around with, so precise are the combinations required for success. One has to learn what these things are too. Although I can throw together a respectable batch of corn bread or most yeast breads with nothing more precise than a mixing bowl and a stirring spoon, I carefully measure all ingredients for biscuits.

In years past, the carbohydrate content of diabetic diets was severely limited. Unless weight control is a problem, carbohydrate is not usually so restricted these days. We have tried to keep most of the bread recipes compatible with low-fat diets. If your carbohydrate restriction is minimal, you should enjoy good eating in this chapter.

Recent evidence has suggested that fiber such as bran has a good effect on the blood sugar. Certainly, fiber has many other advantages. Try the Bran Bread in this chapter for a couple of weeks instead of your usual bread if you are having trouble controlling your diabetes and see what happens.

BRAN MUFFINS

¼ cup wheat germ	¼ cup raisins
¼ cup whole-wheat flour	1 egg, lightly beaten
½ cup bran	½ cup buttermilk
¼ teaspoon salt	1½ tablespoons corn oil
1½ teaspoons baking powder	

Mix all dry ingredients until well blended. Add raisins and continue to mix until raisins are coated. Add egg, milk, and oil and let stand briefly. Oil 6 muffin cups and fill ⅔ full. Bake at 400° for 20 to 30 minutes or well browned. Serves 6.

One muffin contains: 14 grams carbohydrate, 4 grams protein, 6 grams fat, and 125 calories.

Exchange value: 1 muffin = 1 bread and 1 fat.

CORN BREAD MUFFINS

⅓ cup cornmeal, finely ground	¼ teaspoon salt
⅓ cup wheat germ	½ cup buttermilk
⅓ cup whole-wheat flour	1 egg, beaten
1 teaspoon baking powder	

Combine dry ingredients and mix well. Add milk and then egg. Mix well and pour into preheated lightly greased pan. Bake at 375° for about 15 minutes or until well browned. Serves 6.

One muffin contains: 15 grams carbohydrate, 5 grams protein, 3 grams fat, and 106 calories.

Exchange value: 1 muffin = 1 bread.

COMMENT: If much corn bread is eaten, it is important to add some wheat flour, or preferably wheat germ, to the batter, since cornmeal is deficient in several B vitamins that are supplied by wheat. In many parts of the South corn bread may be eaten daily, and in these cases it should certainly be enriched with whole-wheat flours.

This bread is especially good when served with leafy green vegetables. It also complements the flavor of baked or poached fish. It is unsurpassed when served hot with buttermilk or yogurt as an afternoon snack.

SOUTHERN CORN BREAD

Bacon drippings or other fat	1 teaspoon baking powder
½ cup yellow stone-ground cornmeal	½ teaspoon salt
	1 egg
¼ cup wheat germ	½ cup buttermilk
¼ cup flour	2 tablespoons oil

Melt a little bacon drippings or other fat in a heavy skillet or corn bread pan. A cast-iron skillet is good for this. While the skillet and oven are preheating to 425°, combine the other ingredients. If you are using a food processor, put the dry ingredients in and mix briefly. The liquid things can be added together or individually and mixed just enough to blend thoroughly. This can also be done in a blender or by hand. Add the batter to the very hot skillet and bake 15 minutes or until brown but not dry. Serves 6.

(continued)

Total recipe contains: 103 grams carbohydrate, 26 grams protein, 37 grams fat, and 852 calories.

One serving (⅙ of total) contains: 17 grams carbohydrate, 4 grams protein, 6 grams fat, and 142 calories.

Exchange value: 1 serving (⅙ of total) = 1 bread and 1 fat.

PRUNE-NUT BREAD

8 ounces prunes, finely chopped
¼ cup sherry
½ cup chopped walnuts
2 cups whole-wheat flour
¼ cup sugar

½ teaspoon salt
1 teaspoon cinnamon
3 teaspoons baking powder
2 eggs
1 cup buttermilk

Marinate prunes in sherry overnight. Mix the nuts with flour and add other dry ingredients. Mix eggs, buttermilk, prunes, and sherry, and add all at once to the dry ingredients. Bake in a well-greased loaf pan at 350° for 50 minutes or until done in center. Makes 10 slices.

Total recipe contains: 401 grams carbohydrate, 67 grams protein, 56 grams fat, 9 grams alcohol, and 2430 calories.

One slice (1/10 of total) contains: 40 grams carbohydrate, 7 grams protein, 6 grams fat, 1 gram alcohol, and 243 calories

Exchange value: 1 slice (1/10 of total) = 1 fruit, 2 bread, and 1 fat.

SCOTTISH OAT CAKES

1½ cups instant oats
¼ cup cornmeal
¼ cup unsaturated margarine
½ cup whole-wheat flour

½ teaspoon salt
¼ teaspoon baking soda
½ teaspoon baking powder
⅓ cup boiling water

Mix all ingredients except water until thoroughly blended. Add boiling water and stir quickly to mix. Turn out on a floured board, roll about ⅛ to ¼ inch thick, and cut into rounds using a biscuit cutter. Bake on a lightly greased baking sheet at 350° for 30 to 40 minutes. Makes about 10 cakes.

Total recipe contains: 105 grams carbohydrate, 20 grams protein, 48 grams fat, and 830 calories.

One cake (1/10 of total) contains: 10 grams carbohydrate, 2 grams protein, 5 grams fat, and 83 calories.

Exchange value: 1 cake ($\frac{1}{10}$ of total) = 1 bread and 1 fat.

After the first edition of this book was published, Evelyn Villari, who is as close to a sister as I'll ever have, said in all modesty that she had developed a better biscuit recipe than the one I had included. All of my pleadings for the recipe yielded continuing instructions to "take a little butter, about a cup of flour, some salt, and some baking powder," etc.

Finally, it was apparent that there was, in fact, no recipe. She does it like good cooks all over the world. It's called Dump and Stir Cookery. It's also the method I use in my own kitchen when I'm not writing cookbooks! I did finally prevail upon her to measure the biscuits enough times to come up with more precise measurements and that recipe is included herewith.

In the process of all this our charming dietitian, Cathy Paullin, slipped her own recipe for biscuits into the fray. My mother, Irene Middleton, who has made biscuits for breakfast every day of her adult life, thought we were making a bit much of a very simple process and complicated my problem by sending her own recipe (which did not differ from Evelyn's in the casual approach to weights and measures). So developed the Great Biscuit Cookoff. Even with our expert panel of Taster Husbands for judges (we each counted our own votes too), we selected the top four recipes. Since it's my book, I counted my own votes twice and made the following assessment of the products: mine taste best, Mom's are easiest, Evelyn's are most nutritious, and Cathy's are prettiest. There were six dissenting votes for each decision. You'll just have to try them all yourself and decide.

MOM'S BISCUITS

1 cup self-rising flour	$\frac{1}{3}$ cup buttermilk
2 tablespoons pure lard	

Mix all ingredients and roll out on a floured board. Handle as little as possible. Bake on a seasoned cast-iron skillet or other heavy skillet in a 475° oven for 10 minutes or until done. If you don't have self-rising flour on hand, you can use our Pancake Mix (page 40). Makes 12 biscuits.

Total recipe contains: 88 grams carbohydrate, 15 grams protein, 31 grams fat, and 698 calories.

(continued)

One biscuit ($\frac{1}{12}$ of total) contains: 7 grams carbohydrate, 1 gram protein, 3 grams fat, and 58 calories.

Exchange value: 1 biscuit ($\frac{1}{12}$ of total) = $\frac{1}{2}$ bread.

CATHY'S BAKING POWDER BISCUITS

$\frac{1}{2}$ cup plus 1 tablespoon   2 teaspoons sugar
   shortening $\frac{1}{2}$ teaspoon salt
2 cups flour $\frac{1}{2}$ teaspoon cream of tartar
4 teaspoons baking powder $\frac{2}{3}$ cup milk

Cut shortening into dry ingredients. Combine with milk. Knead 8 to 10 times. Roll out $\frac{1}{2}$ inch thick and cut using approximately $2\frac{1}{2}$-inch biscuit cutter. Bake at 400° until done. Makes about 15 biscuits.

Total recipe contains: 211 grams carbohydrate, 32 grams protein, 119 grams fat, and 2025 calories.

One biscuit ($\frac{1}{15}$ of total) contains: 14 grams carbohydrate, 2 grams protein, 8 grams fat, and 135 calories.

Exchange value: 1 biscuit ($\frac{1}{15}$ of total) = 1 bread and $1\frac{1}{2}$ fat.

ANGELA'S BISCUITS

1 cup flour   2 tablespoons margarine
$\frac{1}{2}$ teaspoon salt $\frac{1}{3}$ cup buttermilk
2 teaspoons baking powder

Combine dry ingredients and mix well. Cut margarine in until well mixed. Add buttermilk and quickly turn out on a floured board. Handle as little as possible. Shape into 12 biscuits. Bake on a cookie sheet with biscuits barely touching. Bake at 475° for 10 minutes. Serve immediately with Strawberry Butter (page 164) or Pear Honey (page 163).

Total recipe contains: 88 grams carbohydrate, 15 grams protein, 31 grams fat, and 691 calories.

One biscuit ($\frac{1}{12}$ of total) contains: 7 grams carbohydrate, 2 grams protein, 3 grams fat, and 60 calories.

Exchange value: 1 biscuit ($\frac{1}{12}$ of total) = $\frac{1}{2}$ bread.

EVELYN'S BISCUITS

1 cup flour
1½ teaspoons baking powder
1 tablespoon wheat germ
½ teaspoon salt

¼ teaspoon baking soda
1 tablespoon sweet butter
⅔ cup buttermilk

Mix dry ingredients well. Cut in butter until it is quite fine. Add buttermilk and roll out on a floured board. Bake at 500° for 10 minutes. Makes 12 biscuits.

Total recipe contains: 93 grams carbohydrate, 18 grams protein, 13 grams fat, and 576 calories.

One biscuit (¹/₁₂ of total) contains: 8 grams carbohydrate, 2 grams protein, 1 gram fat, and 48 calories.

Exchange value: 1 biscuit (¹/₁₂ of total) = ½ bread.

ANGELA'S SUNDAY WAFFLES

1 package yeast
½ cup warm milk
1 teaspoon dark molasses
1 egg, separated
¼ teaspoon salt

1 tablespoon oil
¼ cup wheat germ
¼ cup whole-wheat flour
¼ cup chopped pecans
1 tablespoon powdered skim milk

Dissolve yeast in warm milk; add molasses, egg yolk, salt, oil, and wheat germ. Stir until well mixed. Add flour, nuts, and powdered milk. Beat egg white until stiff and fold into batter. Bake on a hot waffle iron. Makes 4 waffles.

Total recipe contains: 56 grams carbohydrate, 30 grams protein, 52 grams fat, and 810 calories.

One serving (½ of total) contains: 28 grams carbohydrate, 15 grams protein, 26 grams fat, and 405 calories.

Exchange value: 1 serving (½ of total) = 2 bread, 1 meat, and 4 fat.

COMMENT: This is a delicious waffle and very nutritious. One serving contains calcium, phosphorus, vitamin E, iron, and B vitamins. Serve with crushed fresh fruit or sugar-free syrup.

The mother of a young child shared the following recipe with me. As any mother knows, children go through stages when they will eat only one thing, or at least it seems like only one thing. Her child was in his "pancake phase." She devised this ingenious method of feeding him properly before school.

THE COMPLETE PANCAKE

1 slice bread	Pinch nutmeg
2 tablespoons evaporated skim milk (or regular whole milk)	1 egg

Put everything in the blender and blend for 30 seconds. Pour out onto a hot griddle. Makes a "short stack." Serves 1 generously, 2 scantily.

Total recipe contains: 18 grams carbohydrate, 13 grams protein, 7 grams fat, and 192 calories.

Exchange value: Recipe = 1 bread and 1½ meat.

COMMENT: This is a nutritionally adequate breakfast for a school-age child if combined with a glass of milk. You could add berries, nuts, wheat germ, brewer's yeast, or whatever you can get away with. Don't forget to add the values for your additives into the calculations.

PANCAKES

⅓ cup whole-wheat flour, sifted	⅓ cup bran
½ teaspoon baking soda	2 tablespoons wheat germ
1 teaspoon baking powder	1 tablespoon oil
¼ teaspoon salt	1 cup buttermilk
⅓ cup quick-cooking oatmeal	1 egg, slightly beaten

Sift first four ingredients together; add remaining dry ingredients and mix well. Mix oil, buttermilk, and egg; add all at once to dry ingredients. Mix well. Bake on nonstick griddle set at medium heat. Makes 10 pancakes.

Total recipe contains: 75 grams carbohydrate, 29 grams protein, 24 grams fat, and 630 calories.

NOTE: Use an equal amount of batter for each pancake. Divide the total figures by the number of pancakes to determine the content of each pancake.

Exchange value: When the recipe is divided into 10 equal-sized pancakes, 2 pancakes may be substituted for 1 bread and 1 fat.

COMMENT: Add leftover corn from the cob, blueberries, sliced bananas, or applesauce, cinnamon, and vanilla to batter for a great special taste. The last one tastes like apple pie. Don't forget to include the added ingredients in your calculations.

EASY PANCAKE

½ cup flour   ½ teaspoon vanilla
½ cup milk   Pinch of nutmeg
2 eggs   ¼ stick butter

Mix all ingredients except butter in a blender or food processor. Melt butter in a glass casserole and add batter. Bake 20 minutes at 425°. Remove from oven and divide into 4 servings. Mix 2 tablespoons lemon juice with artificial sweetener equivalent to 2 tablespoons sugar and sprinkle over pancakes. Serve with applesauce and a dollop of sour cream. Sprinkle with nutmeg. Serves 4.

Total recipe contains: 56 grams carbohydrate, 24 grams protein, 20 grams fat, and 500 calories.

One serving (¼ of total) contains: 14 grams carbohydrate, 6 grams protein, 5 grams fat, and 125 calories.

Exchange value: 1 serving (¼ of total) = ½ bread, ½ whole milk, and 1 fat.

COMMENT: This batter can be kept in the refrigerator for at least a week. A small portion can be cooked in a small round pie plate and used as a crêpe. Omit lemon juice and sweetener and top with a scrambled egg. Garnish with chives or crumbled bacon.

APPLE PANCAKE

1 apple, sliced and unpeeled
1 tablespoon lemon juice
2 tablespoons butter
3 eggs
1 cup milk

1 cup flour
½ teaspoon salt
1 ounce Cheddar cheese,
    shredded

Toss apple and lemon juice and set aside. Divide butter evenly between two rectangular glass baking dishes, about 5 inches by 9 inches, and put in oven to preheat to 500°. Mix remaining ingredients except cheese until well blended. Remove baking dishes from the oven and divide batter equally. Arrange apple slices over top of batter and bake at 500° for 5 minutes. Remove and sprinkle top with cheese. Return to oven, lower temperature to 450°, and bake for 10 minutes. Serves 4.

Total recipe contains: 133 grams carbohydrate, 48 grams protein, 59 grams fat, and 1252 calories.

One serving (¼ total) contains: 33 grams carbohydrate, 12 grams protein, 15 grams fat, and 314 calories.

Exchange value: 1 serving (¼ of total) = 2 bread, 1 meat, and 2 fat.

COMMENT: This dish is complemented by spicy pork sausage or ham.

One of the funny things about writing a cookbook is that all those connected with preparing the manuscript have their own idea about how to make things. For example, our charming typist, Jean Jacob, left a note saying, "I make an apple pancake that is similar but with half the milk and flour." Such a change would, of course, decrease the carbohydrate significantly—so herewith:

APPLE PANCAKE À LA JEAN JACOB

1 apple, sliced
2 tablespoons butter
3 eggs
½ cup flour
½ cup skim milk

Sweetener equivalent to 1
    tablespoon sugar
Cinnamon or powdered sugar
    substitute

Sauté the apple gently in the butter in an 8-inch nonstick skillet. Meanwhile, combine the eggs, flour, milk, and sweetener in a blender. Blend briefly and pour into the hot skillet. Bake in 500° preheated oven for 10 minutes. Sprinkle with cinnamon or powdered sugar substitute. Serves 3.

Total recipe contains: 51 grams carbohydrate, 37 grams protein, 45 grams fat, and 757 calories.

One serving (⅓ of total) contains: 17 grams carbohydrate, 12 grams protein, 15 grams fat, and 278 calories.

Exchange value: 1 serving (⅓ of total) = 1 bread and 2 meat.

CHEESE PANCAKES

½ cup uncreamed cottage cheese
¼ cup evaporated skim milk
½ teaspoon baking powder
1 egg
2 tablespoons white flour

½ pint low-fat yogurt
½ pint strawberries (fresh, canned, or frozen, unsweetened)
Noncalorie sweetener

Blend cheese and milk until smooth. Add baking powder, egg, and flour and blend well. Pour 1 tablespoon of batter for each pancake onto a moderately hot nonstick griddle. When brown on both sides, remove to a hot plate to keep warm. Sweeten strawberries to taste with a noncaloric sweetener. On each pancake place 1 tablespoon strawberries and 1 tablespoon yogurt. Roll the pancake to enclose mixture and serve immediately. Makes 16 pancakes.

Two pancakes contain: 6 grams carbohydrate, 6 grams protein, 2 grams fat, and 60 calories.

Exchange value: 2 pancakes = ½ bread and ½ meat.

Yeast Breads

Many otherwise accomplished cooks confess that a decent loaf of yeast bread is impossible for them to make. If this has been your experience, take the time to measure the temperature in your kitchen in several different spots. If your bread doesn't rise as high and as quickly as you would like, or as the recipe leads you to believe it will, the spot you have chosen is probably too cool. Check it with your thermometer. The ideal spot will be between 80 and 105 degrees. If your dough doesn't rise at all in the chosen places, it is probably too warm. A too warm place will kill the yeast and prevent the bread from rising. The oven is the biggest culprit here. Don't be tempted to set the oven on "warm." That will be too hot. Recipes often recommend putting the dough in a place that is about the temperature of a warm summer day. This is sometimes interpreted to mean in the sun. That also will be too warm. The newest fad in dough management is the microwave oven. Aficionados of this gadget recommend putting the dough in with a container of water and briefly turning on the heat. I haven't tried it myself, but it is said to work well.

You can learn to manipulate the various ingredients in yeast bread to obtain your ideal loaf. Omitting milk and using only water will result in a very crusty loaf. Adding extra fat will yield a finely textured loaf. Brewer's yeast or wheat germ will increase nutritional value. Eggs will add a beautiful golden color.

Since the first edition of this book was published, a new variety of yeast is available. It can be added to the flour, omitting one step in the breadmaking process. Previously, it was necessary to add the yeast to a little warm, sweetened water until it became soft and full of bubbles.

SALLY LUNN

1 package dry yeast	2 tablespoons wheat germ
1 cup white flour	½ teaspoon salt
⅓ cup milk	1 tablespoon sugar
1 egg	2 tablespoons oil

Combine all ingredients and mix thoroughly. Pour into an oiled tube pan. Let rise until doubled in bulk. Bake at 350° for 30 to 45 minutes. Serve hot.

Total recipe contains: 96 grams carbohydrate, 22 grams protein, 20 grams fat, and 652 calories.

One slice (¹⁄₁₀ of total) contains: 10 grams carbohydrate, 2 grams protein, 2 grams fat, and 65 calories.

Exchange value: 2 slices (¹⁄₁₀ of total) = 1½ bread.

BRAN BREAD

2 cups buttermilk	1 cup white flour
3 teaspoons salt	3 cups whole-wheat flour
1 tablespoon molasses	1 cup bran
1 tablespoon yeast	1 cup wheat germ

Mix buttermilk, salt, molasses, yeast, and ½ cup of the white flour. Let stand until bubbly. Add whole-wheat flour and stir 200 times (1 minute in food processor). Let rise until double in bulk. Add bran and wheat germ. Knead in other ½ cup white flour, adding more if necessary to obtain desired consistency. Divide into 3 loaves and let rise in a warm place until doubled in bulk. Bake at 375° for 40 to 45 minutes or until well done. Makes 3 loaves.

Total recipe contains: 475 grams carbohydrate, 114 grams protein, 20 grams fat, and 2540 calories.

One loaf (⅓ of total) contains: 160 grams carbohydrate, 38 grams protein, 7 grams fat, and 850 calories.

Exchange value: 1 slice = 1 bread.

NORWEGIAN BROWN BREAD

1 package yeast
1 cup white flour
3 teaspoons salt
2 cups buttermilk

1 tablespoon molasses
3 cups dark rye flour
3 cups whole-wheat flour
 (preferably stone-ground)

Mix yeast with ½ cup of the white flour and the salt, buttermilk, and molasses. Let stand until bubbly. Add about ½ of the rye and whole-wheat flours and mix well. Cover and let rise in a warm place until about double in bulk. Time will vary according to temperature, but it will take slightly longer than an ordinary bread recipe.

Stir down and add the remainder of the rye and wheat flours. Put the remaining white flour in the kneading bowl and knead until smooth and elastic. This will take 10 to 15 minutes. Slightly more or less flour may be required, depending on the type and texture of the flour. Use additional white flour if it is necessary to add more. Divide into 3 portions and place in well oiled round pans. Allow to rise until doubled again. Bake at 375° for 40 to 45 minutes or until it tests done. Cool on a rack.

Total recipe contains: 600 grams carbohydrate, 130 grams protein, 17 grams fat, and 3073 calories.

One loaf contains: 200 grams carbohydrate, 42 grams protein, 6 grams fat, and 1026 calories.

Exchange value: 1 slice = ½ bread.

COMMENT: Rye bread is my Waterloo, but this recipe yields a delicious crusty loaf with a hearty flavor. It is my husband's favorite brown bread —served warm with butter and a little red wine or black coffee.

PITA BREAD

2½ cups skim milk   6 cups white flour
2 teaspoons salt   1 cup whole-wheat flour
1 package yeast

Mix the milk, salt, and yeast, and add 3 cups of the white flour. Beat at medium speed for 2 minutes. Stir in the whole-wheat flour and then enough of the white flour to make a stiff dough. Use the remaining flour to knead the dough to an elastic consistency. Place in a covered bowl and let rise in a warm place for 1 to 2 hours.

Knead lightly again, just enough to induce the dough to its former volume, and divide into 15 sections. Roll each section into a 6 inch round and place circles on a baking sheet so they do not touch. Bake 10 minutes at 450°.

Cut each round in half and serve with the filling of your choice. These "pocket breads" can be prepared in advance and frozen, if desired. To rewarm, place in a 325° oven for about 5 minutes. Recipe makes 15 rounds, or 30 servings.

Total recipe contains: 610 grams carbohydrate, 106 grams protein, 8 grams fat, and 2936 calories.

One serving (1/30 of total) contains: 20 grams carbohydrate, 3 grams protein, negligible fat, and 100 calories.

Exchange value: 1 serving (1/30 of total) = 1½ bread.

COMMENT: This is an especially good recipe for a low-fat diet.

TOMATO YEAST BREAD

1 package dry yeast   1 tablespoon corn oil
2 cups white flour   1 tablespoon caraway seed
1 teaspoon salt   1 cup rye flour
1 cup tomato juice

Mix yeast with 1 cup of the white flour and salt. Place tomato juice, oil, and caraway seed in a large bowl. Add yeast-and-white-flour mixture.

Stir until free of lumps, then beat for 2 minutes at slow speed on mixer or 200 strokes by hand. Add 1 cup rye flour and mix well. Then add remaining cup of white flour. Dough should be very stiff at this point. Turn out on a floured board and knead until smooth (2 or 3 minutes). Divide into two parts and shape into long narrow loaves. Let rise in a warm (85 to 95°) place until almost doubled in bulk. Bake at 375° for 25 to 30 minutes. Makes 2 loaves.

Total recipe contains: 243 grams carbohydrate, 37 grams protein, 17 grams fat, and 1275 calories.

Exchange value: 1 slice = 1 bread.

Sourdough Breads

Sourdough is the simplest of the yeast breads and is especially useful for low-saturated-fat diets. These breads require the use of sourdough starter (recipe follows), which can be perpetuated indefinitely by a determined housewife. It is customary among sourdough fanciers to give a portion of the starter to friends and neighbors. This friendly gesture is a form of enlightened self-interest. If your starter "goes bad" and you've shared it with many friends, your chances of having the favor returned are much better.

Like all good ideas this can be carried to the extreme. Some years ago my friend Rosemarie Petricelli from the National Institutes of Health was visiting in my home. She became fascinated by the idea of perpetuating a little batch of yeast and wanted some to take back with her to Washington, D.C. We fixed her up a portion and discussed the precautions that were going to be necessary to cope with a few more days in hotels and finally a plane trip from coast to coast. We left out a step somewhere. When Rosemarie arrived home, she had almost a suitcase full of "starter." Makes you wonder how the miners coped!

Between us, Pinkie Ferguson and I have had a batch going continuously for nineteen years!

SOURDOUGH STARTER

1 package yeast	2 cups skim milk
¼ cup warm water	3 cups white flour

Combine yeast and warm water. When dissolved, add to milk and flour. Stir until smooth. Put in a covered glass or plastic container at least 2 quarts in volume. Let rise in refrigerator for several days. When dough is quite spongy and has a pleasant sourdough odor, it is ready to use. Never use all the starter. Always keep 1 cup or more to perpetuate the process. If 1 cup of starter is used, replace with 1 cup of flour and ⅓ cup of skim milk. It can be used daily if replaced in this manner.

One cup of starter contains: 40 grams of carbohydrate, 8 grams of protein, and 0 grams of fat.

Total volume after rising is about 7 cups.

COMMENT: There are many ways to prepare sourdough starter. The best way is to get a portion from a friend. Starters are available commercially and are found in specialty food stores, usually frozen. The above recipe is a compromise to be used when friends and commercial suppliers fail.

PINKIE'S SOURDOUGH HOT CAKES
(from the kitchen of Mary Pinckney Ferguson)

½ cup starter
2 cups warm water
2 cups flour
1 tablespoon sugar
1 teaspoon baking soda

1 teaspoon salt
2 tablespoons boiling water
1 egg
2 tablespoons oil

Place starter in a medium-sized mixing bowl. Add warm water and flour. Beat well and set in a warm place, free from draft, to develop overnight. In the morning the batter will have gained one-half again in bulk and be covered with air bubbles. It will have a yeasty odor. Set aside ½ cup in a refrigerator jar as a starter for next time.

Dissolve sugar, soda, and salt in boiling water. Beat with a fork and blend in egg and oil. Bake on a hot griddle. Serves 6.

One serving (⅙ of total) contains: 33 grams carbohydrate, 6 grams protein, 6 grams fat, and 210 calories.

Exchange value: 1 serving (⅙ of total) = 2 bread and 1 fat.

QUICK SOURDOUGH MUFFINS

½ cup white flour   1 teaspoon baking powder
½ teaspoon salt   ½ cup starter

Combine flour, salt, and baking powder and mix well. Oil a 6-cup muffin tin. Mix starter and dry ingredients. Stir only until well mixed. Drop immediately into tin. Keep volume of muffins about equal. Bake in preheated oven at 425° for 10 to 12 minutes or until well browned. Serve hot with unsaturated margarine or butter. Serves 6.

One muffin contains: 10 grams carbohydrate, 2 grams protein, and 48 calories.

Exchange value: 3 muffins = 2 bread.

COMMENT: These muffins are quickly prepared and are good for breakfast. They are light and very low fat even with added margarine at the table.

NOTE: Measure margarine used for "buttering" and add 4 grams of fat and 36 calories for each teaspoon used.

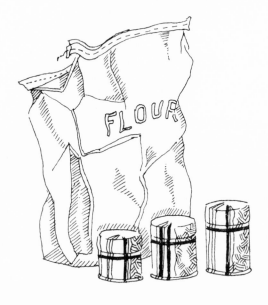

CHAPTER 11

Desserts

- Cheesecake
- Victorian Orange Cake
- Christmas Cake
- Cream Puffs
- Shortcake
- Low-Fat Cheesecake
- Papaya and Blueberries
- Pears with English Cream
- Grapes à la Villa
- Orange Fritters
- Meride Elder's Pineapple Fluff
- Strawberry Sponge
- Froufrou
- Fresh Fruit Whip
- Grapefruit Chiffon
- Peach Parfait
- Fruit Float
- Avocado Dessert
- Holiday Fruit Nog
- Peach Float
- Chocolate-Covered Nuts
- Chocolate Fudge
- Marzipan
- Eggnog Pie
- Huckleberry Pie
- Banana Cream Pie
- Graham Cracker Crust
- Skinny Minnie's Crust
- Walnut Pie Crust
- Oatmeal Cookies
- Chinese Fried Cookies
- Frosted Cookies
- Chocolate Cookies

Just as the first edition of this book went to press, the Food and Drug Administration decided to ban cyclamates for use as artificial sweeteners. That ban destroyed the major part of the dessert section of the first book. There were many recipes that could not be adapted to the use of saccharin, the only remaining sweetener. In desperation, we simply removed the recipes and endured the years of regulatory bargaining that ensued.

Now we find ourselves again going to press while the FDA ponders whether to ban saccharin as well. You will notice that many of the recipes here contain small amounts of sugar. In no case is it enough to cause major changes in the blood sugar, so if the FDA decides to remove saccharin, there will still be some usable recipes left in this section.

Cyclamate had qualities that saccharin does not have. You could both freeze it and cook it without altering the taste and sweetness. Not so with saccharin. Either heating or freezing leaves saccharin tasting everything but sweet. That sad fact severely limits the kinds of dishes that can be prepared using it as a sweetener. So we have reluctantly included some sugar in some recipes. These dishes should not be a regular part of your diet—they are for special occasions.

Canadian readers can still obtain cyclamate but can't get saccharin. Any recipe here can be adapted to the use of cyclamate. We have included the sugar equivalent in most recipes, so just consult the label on your container and include the amount of cyclamate equivalent of that amount of sugar. In most cases it will be equal or close to the amount of saccharin needed.

CHEESECAKE

Crust:

¾ cup quick-cooking rolled oats
½ cup finely chopped walnuts

1 tablespoon butter
2 teaspoons brown sugar

Filling:

3 eggs, separated
¾ cup skim milk
¼ teaspoon salt
2 tablespoons gelatin
1 teaspoon grated lemon peel
2 tablespoons lemon juice
2 teaspoons vanilla

Liquid sweetener equivalent to ¾ cup sugar
1½ pints large-curd creamed cottage cheese
1 cup whipping cream
½ cup powdered milk

Garnish: Chopped nuts or nutmeg

Combine all crust ingredients in a blender or food processor and mix thoroughly. Cover the bottom of an 8- or 10-inch springform pan and bake 5 to 7 minutes in a 350° oven. Cool.

Mix egg yolks, milk, salt, and gelatin and heat in top of double boiler, stirring constantly, until gelatin is well dissolved. Remove from heat when mixture begins to thicken. Stir in lemon peel, juice, vanilla, and liquid sweetener. In a blender or food processor fitted with the steel blade, stir the cottage cheese until very smooth. Fold in the gelatin mixture and chill well. Whip cream and fold into mixture. Beat egg whites until fluffy, adding the powdered milk a tablespoon at a time until it has all been added. Fold the egg whites into the other mixture, pour into the crust, and chill at least 4 hours. Garnish with chopped nuts or nutmeg. Serves 12.

Total recipe contains: 115 grams carbohydrate, 170 grams protein, 192 grams fat, and 2834 calories.

One serving (1/12 of total) contains: 10 grams carbohydrate, 14 grams protein, 16 grams fat, and 236 calories.

Exchange value: 1 serving (1/12 of total) = ½ bread, 2 meat, and 1 fat.

VICTORIAN ORANGE CAKE

½ cup raisins	¾ cup orange juice
1 tablespoon grated orange peel	1 cup flour
½ cup nonfat dry milk	1½ teaspoons baking powder
½ stick butter	½ teaspoon salt
1 egg, beaten	½ cup chopped nuts

Sauce:

1 cup orange juice	1½ teaspoons liquid sweetener
1½ tablespoons dark rum	(equivalent to ½ cup sugar)

Chop raisins finely and add to orange peel. Cream powdered milk with butter. Add the beaten egg and then the orange juice. Mix dry ingredients and combine with the raisin-orange mixture. Combine the dry portion with the liquid and mix well. Stir in nuts and pour batter into an oiled pan. Bake in a preheated oven at 325° for 45 minutes or until it tests done.

Simmer the orange juice and rum for 10 minutes. Remove from heat and cool. Add liquid sweetener.

When cake is cool, transfer to a serving platter. Drizzle the sauce over the top a bit at a time until it is entirely absorbed. Put in refrigerator and leave for at least a day. It improves with age.

Total recipe contains: 232 grams carbohydrate, 44 grams protein, 92 grams fat, 10 grams alcohol, and 2080 calories.

One serving (⅛ of total) contains: 29 grams carbohydrate, 5 grams protein, 11 grams fat, 1 gram alcohol, and 260 calories.

Exchange value: 1 serving (⅛ of total) = 1 fruit, 1½ bread, and 2 fat.

CHRISTMAS CAKE

¼ cup sugar	1 cup coarsely chopped pecans
2 tablespoons margarine	¼ cup white raisins
1 egg	½ cup white flour
2 tablespoons Bourbon	¼ teaspoon baking powder

Cream sugar and margarine. Add egg and Bourbon and beat well. Dredge nuts and raisins with flour. Add baking powder to the rest of the flour and blend with margarine mix; then add nuts and raisins. Mix until just blended. Pour into well-oiled pan and bake at 325° for about 45 minutes or until a toothpick comes out clean. Slice into very thin slices and serve as fruit cake.

Total recipe contains: 131 grams carbohydrate, 23 grams protein, and 103 grams fat.

COMMENT: Dark raisins can be used, but the final cake is not as attractive. Contents must be calculated from weight of finished cake. The maneuvers are as follows:
1. Weigh cake.
2. Divide 131 grams of carbohydrate, 23 grams of protein, and 103 grams of fat by the weight of the cake.
3. Weigh slice to be served the diabetic.
4. Multiply (3) times the product (2). This will give the figures for the diabetic serving.
OR
Divide weight of the slice to be served by weight of the entire cake, and multiply by the figures above to obtain the amount of carbohydrate, protein, and fat in the weighed slice.
Example:
1. Suppose the entire cake weighs 20 ounces.
2. Each slice to be served weighs 2 ounces.
3. 2 ounces divided by 20 ounces = 0.1 (or 1/10th); then 131 grams of carbohydrate × 0.1 = 13.1 grams of carbohydrate, 23 grams of protein × 0.1 = 2.3 grams of protein, and 103 grams of fat × 0.1 = 10.3 grams

of fat. Therefore a 2-ounce serving provides 13.1 grams of carbohydrate, 2 to 3 grams of protein, and 10.3 grams of fat.

CREAM PUFFS

Puffs:

¼ cup unsaturated margarine   Pinch of salt
½ cup boiling water   2 large eggs
½ cup flour, sifted

Filling:

2 egg whites   1 cup strawberries
¼ cup powdered skim milk   Powdered sugar substitute
Liquid sweetener

Cut margarine into small pieces and add to boiling water. Stir to dissolve completely. When mixture is boiling vigorously, add flour and salt. Keep heat low and stir batter rapidly with wooden spoon. When batter pulls away from sides of pan, remove from heat and beat in eggs, one at a time. When well mixed, drop by spoonfuls onto greased cookie sheet, making amount of dough in each as nearly equal as possible. Bake in very hot oven (450°) for 10 minutes. Reduce heat to 400° and continue baking until puffs are firm and brown on top; there should be no beads of moisture on surface (takes about 25 minutes.) Cool on wire rack.

While the puffs are cooling, make the filling. Beat egg whites until they stand in stiff peaks. Add powdered milk, 1 tablespoon at a time, continuing to beat. Add liquid sweetener to taste and then add strawberries. Beat until well mixed and quite stiff.

Cut the cooled puffs in half and fill with an equal amount of filling. Sprinkle each with a teaspoonful of powdered sugar substitute.

1 puff contains: 7 grams carbohydrate, 3 grams protein, 10 grams fat, and 130 calories.

Exchange value: 1 puff = ½ bread and 2 fat.

One filled puff contains: 10 grams carbohydrate, 5 grams protein, 10 grams fat, and 150 calories.

Exchange value: ½ bread, ½ fruit, and 2 fat.

SHORTCAKE

2 cups flour, sifted
2 tablespoons sugar
1 tablespoon baking powder

1 teaspoon salt
6 tablespoons margarine
⅔ cup skim milk

Sift dry ingredients together. Cut in 5 tablespoons of the margarine until fine crumbs form. Add milk and stir lightly. Turn out on floured board and knead smooth. Divide into two parts, and fit one part into 8-inch pie pan. Melt the reserved tablespoon margarine and use it to coat the top of this part. Fit the remaining dough on top and bake at 450° for 15 minutes. Separate the layers when done. Makes 8 servings.

Total recipe contains: 199 grams carbohydrate, 32 grams protein, and 70 grams fat.

1 serving (⅛ of total) contains: 25 grams carbohydrate, 4 grams protein, and 9 grams fat.

COMMENT: Strawberries, blueberries and peaches, raspberries, and so on can be used with this bread for conventional shortcakes. Don't forget to add figures for the fruit and whipped topping, if used, obtaining values from Table 2, p. 12.

LOW-FAT CHEESECAKE

Crust:

¾ cup Grape-nuts
1 tablespoon butter, melted

1 teaspoon brown sugar
1 teaspoon grated orange rind

Filling:

3 eggs, separated
1½ cups skim milk
½ cup nonfat dry milk
1 teaspoon vanilla
Liquid sweetener equivalent to ¾
    cup sugar

2 tablespoons gelatin
3 cups ricotta cheese
1 tablespoon orange juice
1 tablespoon lemon juice
1 teaspoon grated orange rind
1 teaspoon grated lemon rind

Combine Grape-nuts, butter, brown sugar, and orange rind and blend well. Press crumbs onto bottom of a 10-inch pan (preferably springform). Bake in a 350° oven for 5 minutes and cool.

Beat egg yolks and milk; add gelatin and cook in a double boiler until gelatin is dissolved and mixture coats spoon. Chill until mixture is slightly thickened.

Whip ricotta cheese in a blender or a food processor until smooth. Beat egg whites to form peaks and gradually add powdered milk a tablespoon at a time until the whole amount has been added. Beat in the vanilla and liquid sweetener. Add the orange and lemon juices and rind to the ricotta cheese and blend well. Gradually add the egg whites to the chilled gelatin mixture and then combine this mixture with the ricotta. Pour into the springform pan and chill for several hours until quite firm. Makes 12 servings.

Total recipe contains: 151 grams carbohydrate, 148 grams protein, 91 grams fat, and 2049 calories.

One serving (¹⁄₁₂ of total) contains: 13 grams carbohydrate, 12 grams protein, 8 grams fat, and 172 calories.

Exchange value: 1 serving (¹⁄₁₂ of total) = ½ cup milk and 1 medium-fat meat.

PAPAYA AND BLUEBERRIES

2 fresh papayas (180 grams each,   2 ounces blueberries
   prepared)   Powdered sugar substitute
1 lime

Cut papayas into halves lengthwise and scoop out seeds. Remove outer peel. Sprinkle all surfaces with juice of lime. Chill well. When ready to serve, drain excess lime juice into small container. Fill papaya cavities with fresh or frozen blueberries (unsweetened) and sprinkle berries with drained lime juice and powdered sugar substitute. Serves 4.

Total recipe contains: 50 grams carbohydrate, 2 grams protein, 0 grams fat, and 192 calories.

One serving (¼ of total) contains: 12 grams carbohydrate, 48 calories, and vitamins A and C

Exchange value: 1 serving (¼ of total) = 1 fruit.

COMMENT: This is a colorful and tasty dessert. If papaya is not available, cantaloupe or honeydew melon can be substituted. Frozen berries are not nearly as good as fresh but will do. The papayas can be prepared several hours ahead. All desserts should be as easy and nutritious as this.

PEARS WITH ENGLISH CREAM

4 pears	2 lemon twists
1 cup red wine	Liquid sweetener equivalent to 1
2 pieces cinnamon stick	cup sugar

Peel, halve, and core pears. Combine the red wine, cinnamon, and lemon twists in a saucepan and add pears. The liquid should cover the pears completely. Simmer for 10 minutes. Remove from heat, let cool slightly, and add liquid sweetener, turning the pan gently to mix it in without breaking the pear halves apart. Let sit in the liquid while the cream is prepared.

This step can be done in advance if desired, but the pears should be warm when served. Remember, you can't boil it once the sweetener has been added.

English Cream

4 egg yolks	sugar
1 tablespoon flour	1 cup evaporated milk, well
1 cup milk	chilled
1 teaspoon vanilla	2 tablespoons powdered sugar
Liquid sweetener equal to ½ cup	substitute

Mix egg yolks, flour, and milk until smooth. Heat in top of double boiler until thick and smooth, stirring constantly (10 to 15 minutes). Remove from heat and add vanilla and liquid sweetener. Cool thoroughly.

Whip the chilled evaporated milk until soft peaks form. Gradually add the powdered sugar substitute. Fold cream into the custard and cool again.

To serve: lift pears from the poaching liquid and pour the chilled cream over them. Allow ½ pear per serving. Serves 8.

Total recipe, including pears: 166 grams carbohydrate, 44 grams protein, 53 grams fat, and 1390 calories.

One serving (⅛ of total) contains: 20 grams carbohydrate, 7 grams protein, 7 grams fat, and 171 calories.

COMMENT: Canned pears can be used as follows: Drain well. Add to the hot poaching broth. Allow to stand for at least ½ hour.

GRAPES À LA VILLA

½ cup sour half and half   substitute
2 tablespoons brown sugar   1 pound white seedless grapes

Combine the half and half and the brown sugar substitute. Fill 4 tall sherbet glasses with white seedless grapes. Top with the cream topping. Sprinkle with grated nutmeg. Serves 4.

Total recipe contains: 49 grams carbohydrate, 8 grams protein, 17 grams fat, and 358 calories.

One serving (¼ of total) contains: 12 grams carbohydrate, 2 grams protein, 4 grams fat, and 90 calories.

Exchange value: 1 serving (¼ of total) = ½ fruit and 1 fat.

ORANGE FRITTERS

1 large thick-skinned seedless   1 egg, separated
  orange   ⅛ teaspoon cream of tartar
1 teaspoon sugar   1 tablespoon cornstarch
¼ teaspoon nutmeg   Oil for deep frying

Grate enough orange peel to measure at least 1 teaspoonful. Finish peeling the orange, being careful to remove all the white pith. Slice into ½-inch-thick rounds. Place slices on paper towel and sprinkle with 1 teaspoon sugar and nutmeg, mixed.

Beat the egg white until stiff, add cream of tartar, and beat slightly. Add the cornstarch gradually to the stiff egg white. Combine the egg yolk and grated orange rind until well mixed. Gradually fold into the egg white.

Dip the orange slices into the batter and fry one or two at a time in the hot oil for 2 to 3 minutes or until the coating is golden brown. Drain, and serve while hot.

These can be used as a side dish with meat or Chinese food or as a hot dessert. Serves 6.

Total recipe contains: 40 grams carbohydrate, 9 grams protein, 6 grams fat, and 414 calories.

One serving (¼ of total) contains: 7 grams carbohydrate, 1 gram protein, 4 grams fat, and 69 calories.

Exchange value: 1 serving (¼ of total) ½ fruit and 1 fat.

MERIDE ELDER'S PINEAPPLE FLUFF

1 envelope unflavored gelatin
1 can (15 ounces) unsweetened
  crushed pineapple
1 cup evaporated skim milk,
  thoroughly chilled

2 tablespoons lemon juice
¾ teaspoon coconut extract
¾ teaspoon rum extract
Liquid sweetener equivalent to 1
  tablespoon sugar

Combine the gelatin and the liquid drained from the pineapple in a saucepan and heat until completely dissolved. In a large bowl beat the chilled milk and lemon juice until it is the consistency of whipped cream. Add the gelatin mixture, the extracts, and the sweetener. Fold in the drained pineapple. Serves 10.

Total recipe contains: 91 grams carbohydrate, 28 grams protein, ½ gram fat, and 459 calories.

One serving (¹⁄₁₀ of total) contains: 9 grams carbohydrate, 3 grams protein, and 46 calories.

Exchange value: 1 serving (¹⁄₁₀ of total) = 1 fruit.

STRAWBERRY SPONGE

1 envelope unflavored gelatin
½ cup cold water
1 tablespoon liquid sweetener

1½ tablespoons lemon juice
1 pint strawberries, crushed
2 egg whites

Soften gelatin in water in top of double boiler. Add liquid sweetener and lemon juice; heat, stirring until gelatin dissolves. Remove from heat and add crushed berries. Let stand until mixture begins to thicken; then beat until light and fluffy. Beat egg whites until stiff; fold into gelatin mixture. Spoon into six individual molds or into a large 3-cup mold, lightly oiled. Chill until firm. Serves 6.

Total recipe contains: 23 grams carbohydrate, 16 grams protein, 0 grams fat, and 180 calories.

One serving (⅙ of total) contains: 4 grams carbohydrate, 3 grams protein, and 30 calories.

Exchange value: 1 serving (⅙ of total) = ½ fruit.

FROUFROU

1 pint low-fat yogurt   4 tablespoons sugar-free jelly or
                                      jam, any flavor (10 percent
                                      carbohydrate)

Thoroughly mix ingredients and serve in sherbet glasses, well chilled. Serves 4.

Total recipe contains: 34 grams carbohydrate, 16 grams protein, 8 grams fat, and 260 calories.

One serving (¼ of total) contains: 8 grams carbohydrate, 4 grams protein, 2 grams fat, and 65 calories.

Exchange value: 1 serving (¼ of total) = ½ milk.

COMMENT: If fresh fruit and artificial sweetener are used instead of the jelly recommended above, vitamin C and usually vitamin A are added. This is a pleasantly tart dessert that is easy on the calorie counters. It is also a good source of calcium, phosphorus, and B vitamins, especially for people who don't enjoy milk.

FRESH FRUIT WHIP

3 egg whites   Liquid sweetener to taste
¼ cup powdered skim milk   1 cup fresh fruit, crushed

Whip egg whites until they stand in stiff peaks. Add powdered milk, 1 tablespoon at a time. Add liquid sweetener to taste. Add crushed fruit and continue beating at high speed until mixture stands in stiff peaks. Chill in freezer at least 1 hour before serving. Makes 8 servings of ½ cup each.

Total recipe contains: 8 grams carbohydrate, 15 grams protein, 0 grams fat, and 240 calories.

One serving (½ cup) contains: 5 grams carbohydrate, 2 grams protein, and 30 calories if raspberries, strawberries, blackberries, peaches, or apricots are used.

Exchange value: 1 serving (½ cup, or ⅛ of total) = ½ fruit.

COMMENT: This dessert tastes better if the fruit is somewhat tart. Raspberries and apricots both make outstanding desserts. Use whatever is plentiful and alter the calculations according to the amount of fruit used.

GRAPEFRUIT CHIFFON

1 medium grapefruit	¼ cup lemon juice
1½ cups grapefruit juice	¼ teaspoon grated lemon peel
1 package strawberry sugarless dessert mix	¼ teaspoon cream of tartar
	¼ cup powdered skim milk
3 eggs, separated	

Remove grapefruit sections and place in colander to drain. Heat 1 cup of the grapefruit juice to boiling and use to dissolve dessert mix. Beat egg yolks and combine in pan with remaining ½ cup grapefruit juice, lemon juice, and lemon peel; cook over low heat, stirring constantly. When mixture lightly covers spoon, remove from heat and stir into gelatin mixture. Be sure gelatin is completely dissolved. Chill the mixture until it will mound on a spoon but is not solid yet.

Beat egg whites with cream of tartar until frothy; add the powdered skim milk gradually and continue beating until stiff peaks form. Beat gelatin mixture until light and frothy. Fold in grapefruit sections, then egg-white mixture. Put in serving dishes and chill until firm—this will take several hours. Makes 6 servings of ½ cup each.

Total recipe contains: 70 grams carbohydrate, 35 grams protein, 18 grams fat, and 600 calories.

One serving (⅙ of total) contains: 12 grams carbohydrate, 6 grams protein, 3 grams fat, and 100 calories.

Exchange value: 1 serving (⅙ of total) = 1 fruit and 1 meat.

COMMENT: The above combination can also be used as a pie filling. This is not encouraged because of the high fat content of pastry and the enormous increase in calories. For example, if the ½-cup serving recommended above were taken on a slice of average pie crust, the content would be 26 grams carbohydrate, 8 grams protein, 12 grams fat, and 245 calories.

PEACH PARFAIT

½ cup peach purée	Liquid sweetener to taste
2 tablespoons cornstarch	3 ounces Neufchâtel cheese
½ cup water	¼ cup powdered sugar substitute
2 tablespoons lemon juice	4 cups sliced peaches

Combine peach purée, cornstarch, water, and lemon juice. Boil and stir until thick and clear. Add liquid sweetener to taste (you will need about the equivalent of ⅔ cup sugar) and set aside to cool. Blend cheese and powdered sugar substitute until smooth and light. Layer cheese, purée, and peach slices in parfait glasses and chill before serving. If there is a time lag between preparation and serving, sprinkle additional lemon juice over peach slices to prevent browning. Serves 8.

Total recipe contains: 101 grams carbohydrate, 12 grams protein, 20 grams fat, and 680 calories.

One serving (⅛ of total) contains: 13 grams carbohydrate, 2 grams protein, 3 grams fat, and 85 calories.

Exchange value: 1 serving (⅛ of total) = 1 fruit and ½ fat.

COMMENT: The cheese mixture can be stretched by blending several tablespoons of evaporated milk (skim) with it. This also makes it easier to spread in the parfait glasses. Three ounces of cheese will easily blend with ½ cup of evaporated milk. If this amount is used, increase figures for the total recipe by 12 grams carbohydrate, 8 grams protein, and 80 calories. Divide these figures by 8 to get the content of one serving.

FRUIT FLOAT

1 cup strawberries   1 cup whole milk
Liquid sweetener to taste

Blend strawberries in a blender until well puréed. Add sweetener and milk and mix thoroughly. Makes 1 serving.

One serving (total recipe) contains: 23 grams carbohydrate, 8 grams protein, 10 grams fat, and 214 calories.

Exchange value: 1 serving (total recipe) = 1 fruit and 1 milk.

COMMENT: This is an especially good warm-weather drink for children and active adults. It is often successful in getting milk down when other methods fail. It can be made richer by using 1 cup evaporated milk instead of fresh. In this case, double the carbohydrate, protein, and fat contributed by the milk above and increase the milk exchange to 2 instead of 1. This may also be used as part of the emergency diet.

AVOCADO DESSERT

1 large ripe avocado
Juice of 1 lime
Liquid sweetener to taste

Chopped nuts or thin lime slice,
   for garnish

Combine all ingredients and mix in blender until quite smooth. Put in sherbet cups and chill well. Garnish with chopped nuts or thin slice lime. Serves 2 generously.

Total recipe contains: 18 grams carbohydrate, 4 grams protein, and 33 grams fat.

One serving (½ of total) contains: 9 grams carbohydrate, 2 grams protein, 16 grams fat, and 185 calories.

It is obviously not for weight watchers.

Exchange value: 1 serving (½ of total) = 1 fruit and 3 fat.

HOLIDAY FRUIT NOG

2 cups apricot nectar, frozen
2 cups unflavored yogurt

3 eggs
½ teaspoon brandy extract

Combine all ingredients in a blender or food processor. Whirl until smooth. Pour into a serving bowl. Sprinkle with nutmeg. Sweeten with artificial sweetener to taste, if desired. Makes 1 quart, or 8 half-cup servings.

Total recipe contains: 90 grams carbohydrate, 34 grams protein, 24 grams fat, and 668 calories.

One serving (½ cup) contains: 11 grams carbohydrate, 4 grams protein, 3 grams fat, and 87 calories.

Exchange value: 1 serving (½ cup, or ⅛ of total) = ½ fruit and ½ two-percent milk.

PEACH FLOAT

1 medium peach
1 tablespoon lemon juice

¾ cup whole milk
Liquid sweetener to taste

Purée peach and lemon juice in blender. When quite liquid, add milk and liquid sweetener to taste. Mix well and serve immediately.

One serving (total recipe) contains: 20 grams carbohydrate, 6 grams protein, 8 grams fat, and 175 calories

Exchange value: 1 serving (total recipe) = 1 fruit and ¾ milk.

COMMENT: Many fruit combinations can be used, and the calculations are simple. All can be topped with a tablespoon of vanilla ice cream or whipped topping of some kind. If you add this, don't forget to include it in your calculations. This drink may be used as part of an emergency diet.

CHOCOLATE-COVERED NUTS

½ stick butter
6 ounces unsweetened chocolate
2 tablespoons liquid sweetener

½ teaspoon vanilla
8 ounces nut halves

Melt butter and chocolate over low heat. Add other ingredients, except nuts. Remove from heat and add nuts. Drop in clusters on an oiled surface. The nuts can be dipped individually for fancier sweets. They can be redipped when cool for a heavier layer of chocolate. Makes about 1 pound.

Total recipe contains: 85 grams carbohydrate, 44 grams protein, and 282 grams fat.

CHOCOLATE FUDGE

½ stick butter
2 ounces unsweetened chocolate
1 tablespoon liquid sweetener

½ teaspoon vanilla
8 ounces cream cheese, softened
½ cup chopped nuts

Melt butter over low heat. Add chocolate and allow just to melt. Add sweetener and vanilla and remove from heat. In a blender or food processor, quickly mix the melted butter, chocolate, and sweetener with the cream cheese. Stir in the nuts and allow to cool in the refrigerator. This will last about a week in the refrigerator. Makes 20 pieces.

Total recipe contains: 31 grams carbohydrate, 30 grams protein, 199 grams fat, and 2020 calories.

One piece (1/20 of total) contains: 2 grams carbohydrate, 1 gram protein, 10 grams fat, and 101 calories.

Exchange value: 1 piece (1/20 of total) = 2 fats.

MARZIPAN

4 tablespoons butter, softened	½ teaspoon vanilla
4 tablespoons light corn syrup	2 cups powdered sugar substitute
¼ teaspoon salt	8 ounces almond paste
¼ teaspoon almond extract	1 cup nonfat dry milk

Cream butter, gradually adding the corn syrup, salt, almond extract, and vanilla. Alternately add sugar substitute and almond paste. Finally add powdered milk. It should be the consistency of pie dough. Makes 1 pound.

Total recipe contains: 206 grams carbohydrate, 47 grams protein, 118 grams fat, and 4000 calories.

One serving (½ ounce) contains: 6.5 grams carbohydrate, 1.5 grams protein, 3.5 grams fat, and 125 calories.

Exchange value: 1 serving = 1 bread and 1½ fat.

EGGNOG PIE

3 eggs, separated	1½ tablespoons rum
½ cup powdered skim milk	1 cup heavy cream
1½ teaspoons liquid sweetener	1 envelope unflavored gelatin
(equivalent to ½ cup sugar)	1 teaspoon vanilla
1½ tablespoons brandy	Graham Cracker Crust (page 159)

Beat yolks and add dry milk, and liquid sweetener. Add brandy and rum and continue beating. Soften gelatin in water and heat until completely dissolved. Add egg-yolk mixture. Beat egg whites until stiff. Whip cream until it stands in peaks and add vanilla. Fold whites and cream together and blend with egg-yolk mixture. Pour into a graham cracker crust and chill for several hours. Sprinkle top with nutmeg before serving. Serves 8 to 10.

Total filling contains: 24 grams carbohydrate, 43 grams protein, 107 grams fat, and 15 grams alcohol.

Total crust contains: 199 grams carbohydrate, 29 grams protein, 70 grams fat, and 1542 calories.

One piece (⅛ total pie) contains: 26 grams carbohydrate, 11 grams protein, 23 grams fat, 2 grams alcohol, and 369 calories.

Exchange value: 1 piece (⅛ pie) = 1 bread, 1 medium-fat meat, and 3 fat.

HUCKLEBERRY PIE

1 envelope unflavored gelatin
¼ cup cold water
½ cup puréed huckleberries
1½ cups whole huckleberries
2 cups evaporated milk,
  thoroughly chilled

Liquid sweetener equivalent to ¾
  cup sugar
1 tablespoon lemon juice
1 teaspoon vanilla
Baked Pie Crust (page 90) (use
  half recipe)

Soften gelatin in cold water. Add to the puréed huckleberries. Heat until gelatin dissolves. Stir in the remaining berries and chill. Whip the milk and add the liquid sweetener, lemon juice, and vanilla. Fold into the berry mixture. Pour into a baked pie crust and chill 3 to 4 hours. Serves 8.

Total recipe contains: 93 grams carbohydrate, 46 grams protein, 41 grams fat, and 916 calories.

One serving (⅛ pie) contains: 12 grams carbohydrate, 6 grams protein, 5 grams fat, and 114 calories.

Exchange value: 1 serving (⅛ pie) = ½ whole milk and ½ fruit.

BANANA CREAM PIE

3 eggs
Dash of salt
½ cup evaporated skim milk
1¼ cups fresh skim milk
Powdered sweetener equivalent to
  ½ cup sugar

¾ teaspoon vanilla
1 cup sliced bananas
1 tablespoon lemon juice
9-inch Graham Cracker Crust
  (page 159)

Beat eggs with salt and evaporated milk until well mixed. Add fresh milk and powdered sweetener. Cook in top of double boiler until mixture is consistency of soft custard. Add vanilla, mix well, and remove from heat. Toss sliced bananas with lemon juice and arrange in bottom of graham cracker crust, reserving several slices for garnish. Pour custard mix over the bananas. Arrange reserved slices over the top and chill until set.

COMMENT: The basic recipe can be used for almost any cream pie. For coconut cream pie, use 1½ cups freshly grated coconut or unsweetened coconut (found in health food stores) instead of the bananas. Mix 1 cup of the coconut with the cream base and use the remaining coconut to garnish the top. Those who can have saturated fat only in extremely limited amounts should not use the variation because of the high saturated-fat content of coconut.

GRAHAM CRACKER CRUST

1½ cups fine graham cracker   4 tablespoons margarine
   crumbs

Mix well and press into 9-inch pie plate. Use another plate of equal size to pack crumbs in firmly. Chill or freeze until ready to use. Serves 8.

One slice (⅛ of crust) contains: 22 grams carbohydrate, 7 grams protein, 16 grams fat, and 260 calories.

Exchange value: 1 slice (⅛ of crust) = 1 bread, ½ milk, and 2 fat.

SKINNY MINNIE'S CRUST

2 tablespoons shortening   2 tablespoons ice water
½ cup bran   ¼ teaspoon salt
½ cup flour   ¼ teaspoon baking powder

Melt shortening and add to bran. Mix thoroughly. Put into freezer for at least ½ hour. Combine other ingredients to form a ball and add bran-margarine mixture. Roll out lightly on pastry cloth. Fit into a pie plate and bake at 350° until lightly browned. Serves 8.

Total recipe contains: 63 grams carbohydrate, 9 grams protein, 29 grams fat, and 541 calories.

One serving (⅛ of total) contains: 8 grams carbohydrate, 1 gram protein, 4 grams fat, and 68 calories.

Exchange value: 1 serving (⅛ of total) = ½ bread and 1 fat.

WALNUT PIE CRUST

1 cup quick-cooking rolled oats   ⅓ cup melted diet margarine
¾ cup chopped walnuts

Toast the oats in a 325° oven for 10 minutes. Remove and combine with the other ingredients. Press into a 9-inch pie tin, using another pie tin of equal size to pack the crust in firmly. Chill before filling. Can be frozen. Serves 8.

Total recipe contains: 72 grams carbohydrate, 25 grams protein, 96 grams fat, and 1185 calories.

One serving (⅛ of total) contains: 9 grams carbohydrate, 3 grams protein, 12 grams fat, and 148 calories.

Exchange value: 1 serving (⅛ of total) = ½ bread and 2½ fats.

OATMEAL COOKIES

1½ cups quick-cooking oatmeal   2 teaspoons baking powder
⅔ cup margarine, melted   ½ cup skim milk
4 egg whites, slightly beaten   1 teaspoon vanilla
½ cup sugar   ½ cup raisins
1½ cups sifted flour   ½ cup chopped walnuts
½ teaspoon salt

Mix oatmeal and margarine. Blend in egg whites and sugar. Add dry ingredients alternately with milk and vanilla. Add raisins and nuts. Drop by level tablespoons on cookie sheet. Bake in hot (375°) oven for 10 to 15 minutes. Makes about 4 dozen.

Total recipe contains: 381 grams carbohydrate, 63 grams protein, and 170 grams fat.

If an equal amount is used for each cookie, the content of one cookie can be determined by dividing the total figures by the number of cookies.

CHINESE FRIED COOKIES

3 eggs, beaten   1 tablespoon baking powder
1 cup flour   Powdered sugar substitute
⅓ cup sesame seeds, toasted   Oil for deep frying

Combine first 4 ingredients. Roll out to about ⅛-inch thickness. Cut into desired shapes and deep-fry until brown. When slightly cooled sprinkle with sugar substitute. Can be served hot or cold. Will make 1 dozen medium-sized cookies.

Total recipe contains: 97 grams carbohydrate, 45 grams protein, 115 grams fat, and 1656 calories.

One cookie (¹/₁₂ of total) contains: 8 grams carbohydrate, 4 grams protein, 10 grams fat, and 138 calories.

Exchange value: 1 cookie (¹/₁₂ of total) = ½ bread and 2 fat.

FROSTED COOKIES

Cookies:

1 cup diet margarine   2 cups flour
1 cup small-curd cottage cheese

Frosting:

½ cup diet margarine   ⅛ teaspoon salt
Sugar substitute to equal 1⅔ cups   ½ teaspoon vanilla
  powdered sugar
1 tablespoon cocoa

Combine the 1 cup margarine and cheese in a mixer bowl or food processor and mix until smooth and creamy. Gradually add the flour and beat until smooth. Roll out and cut into rounds. Bake on an ungreased cookie sheet for 15 minutes at 350°.

Cream the other ingredients until they are thoroughly mixed and top each cookie with a small dollop.

Makes about 4 dozen cookies.

Total recipe contains: 177 grams carbohydrate, 54 grams protein, 109 grams fat, and 1728 calories.

Two cookies contain: 7 grams carbohydrate, 2 grams protein, 4 grams fat, and 72 calories.

Exchange value: 2 cookies = ½ bread and 1 fat.

CHOCOLATE COOKIES

¼ cup evaporated milk
4 tablespoons butter
½ teaspoon vanilla
Liquid sweetener equivalent to 1
    cup of sugar

2 tablespoons cocoa
½ cup toasted wheat germ
½ cup finely chopped toasted
    almonds or other nuts

Combine milk and butter and heat gently until butter melts. Add vanilla and sweetener and mix well. Remove from heat, add cocoa, and stir until well dissolved. Add wheat germ and nuts and mix well. Drop on oiled plate and let cool. Makes 1 dozen.

Total recipe contains: 46 grams carbohydrate, 33 grams protein, 98 grams fat, and 1200 calories.

One cookie contains: 4 grams carbohydrate, 3 grams protein, 8 grams fat, and 100 calories.

Exchange values: 1 cookie = ⅓ whole milk and 1 fat; 1 cookie and ½ cup milk = 1 whole milk.

COMMENT: These make great after-school treats because of their high nutritive content. Serve with a glass of milk.

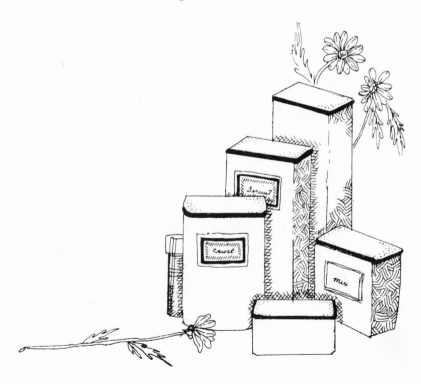

CHAPTER 12

Jellies and Syrups

- **Pear Honey**
- **Strawberry Jam**
- **Strawberry Butter**
- **Fresh Strawberry Jam**
- **Orange Marmalade**

- **Cranberry-Orange Relish**
- **Grape Jelly**
- **Cranberry Sauce**
- **Fresh Mint Jelly**

There are many excellent sugar-free jellies, jams, and syrups available commercially, and unless large amounts are eaten it is probably as economical to buy as to make them. Since sugar-free jellies must be refrigerated, make only as much as will be used in a week or two. The juices can, of course, be frozen when available and thawed for later use.

PEAR HONEY

Lemon wedge (about ⅛ of a
   lemon)
1 cup chopped pear

1 tablespoon water
Liquid sweetener equivalent to ¾
   cup sugar

Seed the lemon and put through the food grinder, blender, or processor. Combine with chopped pear and water and simmer over very low heat until pear becomes very liquid and transparent. The mixture should be about the consistency of thick honey. Remove from heat and cool slightly. Add liquid sweetener. Store in sterilized jar in the refrigerator. Serve with biscuits, waffles, and the like. Makes about 1 cup.

Treat as "free" for normal-size serving.

STRAWBERRY JAM

4 cups berries
1 cup water
1 package Slim-Set (sugar-free

pectin)
Liquid sweetener equivalent to ½
cup sugar

Combine berries, water, and Slim-Set. Heat to boiling in a large kettle and boil vigorously for 2 full minutes. Remove from heat. Skim foam and discard. Let cool slightly and add liquid sweetener. Mix well. Taste for sweetness, adding more sweetener if desired. Pour into sterilized jars or glasses and seal with paraffin wax. Refrigerate after opening. DO NOT FREEZE. Makes 4 cups jam.

Treat as "free" when using average serving sizes.

STRAWBERRY BUTTER

3 tablespoons powdered sugar
    substitute
½ cup butter or margarine,

softened
¼ cup puréed fresh strawberries
(can be frozen)

Cream sugar substitute and butter until light and fluffy. Fold in puréed strawberries. This is great on biscuits, pancakes, and waffles and can be used instead of butter and syrup. It keeps a week or so in the refrigerator. Makes ¾ cup (12 tablespoons).

Total recipe contains: 4 grams carbohydrate, 10 grams protein, 91 grams fat, and 864 calories.

One tablespoon (¹⁄₁₂ of total) contains: 8 grams fat and 72 calories.
Exchange value: 1 tablespoon (¹⁄₁₂ of total) = 1½ fat.

FRESH STRAWBERRY JAM

2½ cups fresh strawberries (or
    frozen dry pack)
2 tablespoons lemon juice

1 teaspoon cornstarch
Liquid sweetener equivalent to ⅓
cup sugar

Combine all ingredients except sweetener in a saucepan and simmer for 20 minutes, stirring frequently. Skim any foam that has accumulated and discard. Remove from heat and cool slightly. Add liquid sweetener ½ teaspoon at a time, tasting after each addition until desired sweetness is reached. Store in refrigerator. This jam will not freeze successfully. Makes 2 cups.

If you wish to preserve berries for jam later in the season, berries can be placed on a cookie sheet in a single layer and frozen. When completely frozen, remove and store in a plastic bag or other bulk container. They can then be removed in whatever quantity is needed later in the season.

ORANGE MARMALADE

Zest from 1 orange
Juice of 2 oranges or 1 cup
  orange juice
½ teaspoon gelatin

Liquid sweetener equivalent to 3
  tablespoons sugar
1 teaspoon lemon juice

Shred the orange peel into fine strips (the juice and peel can be combined in a food processor and chopped finely using the steel blade and alternating cycle). Combine with the juice and gelatin and simmer on low heat for 10 minutes. Remove from heat and cool slightly. Mix the liquid sweetener and lemon juice and add to the orange juice mixture. Cool in refrigerator until thickened.

This can be considered a "free" food in the usual amounts.

CRANBERRY-ORANGE RELISH

2 medium oranges, quartered and
  seeded
½ cup roughly chopped walnuts
1 pound fresh or frozen

cranberries
Liquid sweetener, equivalent to 2
  cups sugar

Chop oranges, nuts, and cranberries finely in the food processor or in a food chopper. Add sweetener and refrigerate. Serve with turkey and dressing or use to fill pear halves for a fruit salad. Makes 1 quart.

This can be considered a "free" food in usual amounts.

GRAPE JELLY

4 cups unsweetened grape juice
1 package Slim-Set (sugar-free
  pectin)

Liquid sweetener equivalent to ½
  cup sugar

Boil juice and Slim-Set for 1 minute. Set aside. Skim foam and discard. Add liquid sweetener. Taste and add more sweetener if desired. Pour into jelly glasses and seal with ¼ inch liquid paraffin on top. DO NOT FREEZE. Makes about 1 quart.

Total recipe contains: 280 grams carbohydrate, 6 grams protein, 0 grams fat, and 1140 calories.

One tablespoon contains: 4 grams carbohydrate, 0 grams protein, 0 grams fat, and 18 calories.

Exchange value: 1 tablespoon = ½ fruit.

CRANBERRY SAUCE

1 pound fresh or frozen
  cranberries
¼ cup water

2 packages unflavored gelatin
Liquid sweetener equivalent to 2
  cups sugar

Combine berries, water, and gelatin and cook gently, stirring frequently, in a saucepan until the berries have popped and gelatin is dissolved. Remove from heat, cool slightly, and add sugar substitute. Pour into a mold and refrigerate until quite firm. Serve with the traditional Thanksgiving meal. Makes 1 quart.

In normal serving amounts I would count this as a "free" food.

FRESH MINT JELLY

1 cup fresh mint leaves
½ cup apple cider vinegar
1 cup water
1 tablespoon gelatin

½ bottle pectin
4 drops green color
Liquid sweetener equivalent to
  3½ cups sugar

Combine the mint, vinegar, water, and gelatin and boil for 30 minutes. Add pectin and color and boil again briefly. Remove from heat, cool slightly, add sweetener, and strain into clean jars. Store in refrigerator.

Makes 2 pints.

For average serving, count as "free."

COMMENT: Serve with fresh lamb.

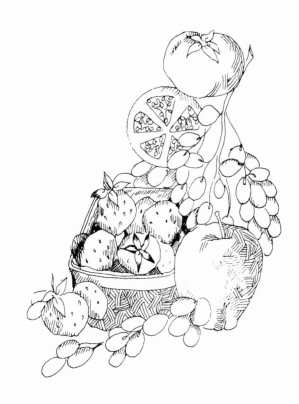

CHAPTER 13

Emergency Diets

- **Liquid No. 1**
- **Liquid No. 2**
- **Liquid No. 3**
- **Liquid No. 4**
- **Special Oatmeal**

- **Enriched Milk Toast**
- **Plain Custard**
- **Blackberry Gelatin**
- **Gelatin Dessert**

A time will inevitably come when your regular diet cannot be consumed. The occasion may be a case of the flu, dental work, or simply poor appetite. The diabetic must keep his intake fairly constant or serious complications may arise. If vomiting or diarrhea occurs, supplemental feedings are necessary, and although management of these illnesses must be supervised by a physician, you should know of liquid formulas that can be taken in an emergency. An adult needs at least a 100 grams of carbohydrate and 30 grams of protein daily when ill. The suggestions that follow can be supplemented with fruit juices, ginger ale, and similar beverages. Generally, citrus juices are not well tolerated when nausea is present, and juices such as blackberry and cranberry are useful to have on hand for such occasions. Recipes for two useful drinks, Fruit Float and Peach Float, are given on pages 154 and 155.

LIQUID NO. 1

1 quart whole milk
2 eggs, well beaten
½ can (6 ounces) orange juice
concentrate

½ cup powdered skim milk

Mix well in blender or jar and use as frequent small feedings. Total volume: 1¼ quarts.

Total recipe contains approximately: 130 grams carbohydrate, 63 grams protein, 46 grams fat, and 1200 calories.

Exchange value: total recipe = 4 bread, 6 meat, 2 whole milk, and 5 fruit.

LIQUID NO. 2

1½ quarts water	2 eggs
2 cups nonfat dry milk	½ cup orange juice

Mix well and serve in divided portions. Total volume: 1¾ quarts.

Total recipe contains: 75 grams carbohydrate, 60 grams protein, 12 grams fat, and 650 calories.

Exchange value: total recipe = 5 skim milk, 2 meat, and 1 fruit.

COMMENT: Skim milk (1½ quarts) can be substituted for the powdered milk and water without unduly affecting the calculations.

LIQUID NO. 3

1 quart whole milk	2 eggs
1 can (6 ounces) evaporated milk	½ cup vanilla ice cream
2 tablespoons brandy or Bourbon	Nutmeg to taste

Blend well and serve in divided portions.

Total recipe contains: 82 grams carbohydrate, 64 grams protein, 68 grams fat, and 1270 calories (73 calories are from alcohol).

Exchange value: total recipe = 5½ milk, 2 meat, 1 bread, and 1 fat.

LIQUID NO. 4

2 tablespoons plain gelatin	1 cup tomato juice
1 quart Chicken Stock (page 73), canned chicken broth, or Beef Stock (page 70)	Salt to taste

Soften gelatin in small amount of cold stock; then add the remaining stock and heat to boiling. Add tomato juice and salt. This can be served as a clear soup along with one of the other liquid diets. It does not fulfill an entire day's nutritional requirements alone.

Total recipe contains: 10 grams carbohydrate, 35 grams protein, and 180 calories.

Additional carbohydrate can be taken as crackers or toast along with this if it is served as a soup. The above calculations are made on the basis of homemade stock. If bouillon cubes are used, increase added gelatin to 4 tablespoons and leave calculations as they appear.

I once scolded a young German mother for feeding her small son only oatmeal for breakfast. She revealed the following combination to me, and I readily admitted that her version of oatmeal was a satisfactory breakfast. I have since recommended it many times to young and old alike who prefer cereals to more substantial breakfast fare.

SPECIAL OATMEAL

1 cup water
2 tablespoons (15 grams) raisins
½ cup (40 grams) oatmeal

½ cup evaporated skim milk
1 egg, well beaten

Use salted water to cook raisins and oatmeal in the usual way. Combine milk and egg and add to cooked oatmeal. Remove from heat and stir until well mixed. Cover and let stand for 5 minutes. Add liquid sweetener to taste and sprinkle with cinnamon. Makes 1 large or 2 smaller servings.

Total recipe contains: 49 grams carbohydrate, 21 grams protein, 9 grams fat, and 361 calories.

Exchange value: total recipe = 1 skim milk, 1 meat, 1 fruit, and 2 bread.

COMMENT: If your allowance of saturated fat is extremely limited, omit the egg yolk and use instead 2 egg whites and 1 teaspoon unsaturated margarine.

ENRICHED MILK TOAST

1 cup whole milk	1 slice dry whole-wheat toast
1 egg, well beaten	Dash of nutmeg

Combine milk and egg; heat gently or in double boiler until steaming hot. Do not boil. Place toast in flat-bottomed bowl and add hot milk-and-egg mixture. Sprinkle with nutmeg.

Total recipe contains: 27 grams carbohydrate, 17 grams protein, 16 grams fat, and 320 calories.

Exchange value: total recipe = 1 bread, 1 whole milk, and 1 meat.

COMMENT: This can also be used for fussy breakfast eaters. It is a painless way to get an egg down a child who temporarily refuses it.

PLAIN CUSTARD

¼ cup sugar	3 eggs (or 3 egg whites and 3
½ cup nonfat dry milk	teaspoons unsaturated
Pinch salt	margarine)
½ cup evaporated skim milk	1½ cups liquid skim milk
1 teaspoon vanilla	

Mix all ingredients except liquid skim milk; beat until smooth. Add skim milk. Pour into four individual baking dishes and sprinkle with nutmeg. Measure or weigh so dishes are of equal volume. Set baking dishes in a pan with small amount of water and bake at 325° until custard is well set on outside, but still soft in center.

Total recipe contains: 86 grams carbohydrate, 45 grams protein, 18 grams fat, and 700 calories.

One serving (¼ of total) contains: 21 grams carbohydrate, 11 grams protein, 5 grams fat, and 175 calories.

Exchange value: 1 serving (¼ of total) = 1 meat and ¾ skim milk.

BLACKBERRY GELATIN

2 cups blackberry juice (canned or	1 package (1 tablespoon) plain
prepared from fresh	gelatin
blackberries, unsweetened)	Liquid sweetener to taste

Heat 1 cup blackberry juice to boiling and use to dissolve gelatin. When completely dissolved, add remaining juice and artificial sweetener to taste. Measure into 4 equal servings.

Total recipe contains: 36 grams carbohydrate, 8 grams protein, 0 grams fat, and 184 calories.

One serving (¼ of total) contains: 9 grams carbohydrate, 2 grams protein, and 44 calories.

Exchange value: 1 serving (¼ of total) = 1 fruit.

COMMENT: This is especially kind to upset stomachs and is often tolerated when other fruits and juices are not. Cranberry juice can be substituted for the blackberry juice without detriment to flavor. Cranberry juice can be purchased in an artificially sweetened form, and if that is used, omit additional sweetener. Two cups dietetic cranberry juice contain 8 grams of carbohydrate; a ½ cup serving of this cranberry gelatin can be taken as a "free" food.

GELATIN DESSERT

1 package sugarless strawberry
  dessert mix
1 cup boiling water

1 cup cool water
1 cup fresh strawberries, whole

Dissolve gelatin in boiling water. Add cool water. Measure into four equal portions. Weigh or measure strawberries and divide into 4 equal portions; add to gelatin and refrigerate until set. This is a very pretty dish and will tempt timid appetites.

Total recipe contains: 11 grams carbohydrate, 6 grams protein, 0 grams fat, and 72 calories.

One serving (¼ of total) contains: 3 grams carbohydrate, 1 gram protein, and 18 calories.

Exchange value: 1 serving (¼ of total) = ⅓ fruit.

CHAPTER 14

Creating Recipes

Most new recipes are created in the test kitchens of companies that have products to sell. Many of these products are excellent, as are the recipes that promote their use. However, some leave much to be desired nutritionally. It is wise to look at new recipes with nutrition in mind and attempt to alter them, if necessary, to increase their value. This is especially important for the diabetic. A new recipe for use in a family with a diabetic member should be evaluated in terms of its content of sugar, total carbohydrate, fat, and vitamins and minerals, and altered as necessary.

ALTERING SUGAR CONTENT

A recipe's sugar content is perhaps its most important feature, since any recipe requiring more than a tablespoon of sugar has to be altered for a diabetic. The various artificial sweeteners have already been considered in Chapter 4. These substances may be used in many recipes but, unfortunately, are not suitable for many others. All companies that sell artificial sweeteners publish small cookbooks that are free for the asking. These booklets contain recipes for the kinds of dishes for which the manufacturer's product is suitable. Compare your recipe with theirs, and if you find a similar one, chances are that yours can be adapted successfully. Most of these manufacturers retain consulting home economists or dietitians who will render opinions on recipes submitted to them.

ALTERING CARBOHYDRATE CONTENT

Not only sugar but total carbohydrate must be considered in new recipes. If the basic materials are flour, potatoes, macaroni, noodles, or similar foods, the carbohydrate content is high. This does not mean that the dish cannot be used but rather that it must be used instead of bread or in very limited quantities. If it is to be substituted for bread, consider the vitamin and mineral content as well. If it does not compare favorably with the content of whole-grain bread, then either alter the recipe by adding an egg for some of the liquid or add a few tablespoons of powdered milk. Added wheat germ will provide extra B vitamins, protein, and trace minerals and is usually undetectable in the final product. As discussed earlier, it is often possible to increase both the vitamin and the mineral content of flours and flour products by adding brewer's yeast to the flour before sifting and measuring. Be sure the flavor of the yeast will be compatible if you are adding much. The amounts of the various vitamins you are adding can be calculated from the information on the yeast box, if you are at all talented in mathematics.

Portions of flour used in pie crusts, pastries, and so on can be replaced with soy flour. This reduces the carbohydrate content and raises the protein level. A light hand is sometimes necessary, however, for if much soy flour is used you may need help to lift the result. A cake baked of even half soy flour is a very heavy cake. On the other hand, soy flour does not detract from the breads one expects to have a heavy texture, and pie crust made entirely from soy flour is respectable indeed.

ALTERING FAT CONTENT

Not only total fat content but the kind of fat must be evaluated. One can almost always replace saturated with unsaturated fat with little detriment to the final result. Egg yolk can be replaced by another egg white and oil. If the egg color is needed, yellow food coloring can be added. Unsaturated margarine can be substituted for butter, low-fat yogurt for sour cream, Neufchâtel cheese for cream cheese (the former contains saturated fat, but less of it). If the total fat content must be reduced, gradually cut down the total amount until the minimal acceptable level has been reached. If you do this each time you prepare a recipe, you can greatly reduce the total amount in many recipes. The low-calorie margarines now on the market help in this regard. Unfortunately, they are not really suitable for frying foods, because of the thickening agents in them, but they make a very tasty substitute for butter on bread, pancakes, and the like. In general, they contain about half as much fat as regular margarine.

ALTERING VITAMIN AND MINERAL CONTENT

Almost any published recipe is the better for this kind of alteration. Some recipes seem to be calculated to give the least nutrition possible! Improvements can be effected by saving the cooking liquid for use in other dishes, substituting a nutritious meat stock for the liquid specified, using less volume of liquid, avoiding soaking and peeling vegetables and fruits, shortening the cooking time, and substituting more nutritious ingredients for some of those specified (for example, whole-grain for refined flour, milk for water).

CALCULATING NUTRITIONAL CONTENT

To calculate the nutritional content of a recipe, you need a good set of food-content lists, similar to but more complete than those in Table 2 of this book. You can obtain a set of food-content lists from your county agent or from the Superintendent of Documents, U.S. Government Printing Office, Washington, D.C. 20402. Single copies are free. Ask for House and Garden Bulletin No. 72, Nutritive Value of Foods. Perhaps your local home economist will explain the calculation procedure to you or suggest other publications that will.

The several examples of nutrition calculations presented earlier in this book should be referred to for exercises. As another example, let us consider the following recipe:

BISCUITS

2 cups flour   ⅓ cup butter
1 tablespoon baking powder   ¾ cup whole milk
1 teaspoon salt

We note that the basic materials are high in carbohydrate and fat content. This can be ameliorated by using whole-wheat flour to provide more vitamins and minerals per gram of carbohydrate and by substituting unsaturated for the saturated fat and skim milk for the whole milk. We now consult the food-content lists for nutritional content of the ingredients. The 2 cups of whole-wheat flour contain 170 grams of carbohydrate, 32 grams of protein, and 4 grams of fat. The ⅓ cup of unsaturated margarine (substituted for the butter) contains 61 grams of fat and negligible carbohydrate and protein. The ¾ cup of skim milk contains 9 grams of carbohydrate, 6 grams of protein, and no fat. The seasonings can be disregarded in this case. Now we add the figures for each ingredient to obtain the total contained in the recipe:

	C	P	F
Flour	170	32	4
Margarine			61
Milk	9	6	
Total	179	38	65

This amount makes one dozen biscuits. If we divide the above totals by the total number of biscuits, we can determine the nutritional content of each biscuit—assuming, of course, that the biscuits are equal in size, and care must be taken in this regard. Each biscuit has the following nutritional content:

$$179/12 = 15 \text{ grams of carbohydrate}$$
$$38/12 = 3 \text{ grams of protein}$$
$$65/12 = 5 \text{ grams of fat}$$

Each biscuit equals 1 bread exchange and 1 fat exchange.

To calculate the calorie content, remember that carbohydrate and protein each contain 4 calories per gram and fat contains 9 calories per gram. The necessary mathematics are as follows:

$$15 \times 4 = 60 \text{ carbohydrate calories}$$
$$3 \times 4 = 12 \text{ protein calories}$$
$$5 \times 9 = 45 \text{ fat calories}$$

Thus there is a total of 117 calories per biscuit. If extra fat is used to "butter" the biscuit, it must be counted in addition.

Although these mechanics seem complicated to the beginner, if used frequently they will become second nature. When the method is mastered completely, the nutritional content of any recipe can be determined and the new dish introduced with no detriment to the diabetic diet.

FOOD SUBSTITUTES

"What about 'artificial foods'?" is a question often asked. In general, I am not keen about food substitutes, but they are useful in certain situations. The egg substitutes permit preparation of many dishes that would be impossible for patients on low-cholesterol diets. The diet margarines give the illusion of butter for people on low-fat diets. The artificial creams have little to recommend them, as they contain saturated fat and therefore have only the decreased cholesterol in their favor. There are many whipped toppings that are artificially sweetened that may be useful to substitute for whipped cream if cholesterol intake is limited. They too contain fat, so are not of too much value when total fat intake is limited.

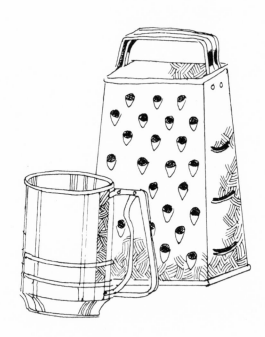

TABLE OF METRIC EQUIVALENTS
(Volume and Weight)

Volume (common units)

1 ounce	28.35 grams
1 pound	453.59 grams
1 gram	0.035 ounces
1 kilogram	2.21 pounds

Weight (common units)

1 cup	16 tablespoons
	8 fluid ounces
	236.6 milliliters
1 tablespoon	3 teaspoons
	0.5 fluid ounce
	14.8 milliliters
1 teaspoon	4.9 milliliters
1 liter	1,000 milliliters
	1.06 quarts
1 bushel	4 pecks
1 peck	8 quarts
1 gallon	4 quarts
1 quart	2 pints
1 pint	2 cups
	473.2 milliliters

AFFILIATE DIABETES ASSOCIATIONS
AND COMPONENT ORGANIZATIONS

ALABAMA

American Diabetes Association
Alabama Affiliate, Inc.
  904 Bob Wallace Avenue, S.E., Suite
  222
  Huntsville, Alabama 35801

ALASKA

See Washington Affiliate.

ARIZONA

Arizona Diabetes Association, Inc.
  555 West Catalina Drive, #14
  Phoenix, Arizona 85013
Tucson Unit
  4901 E. Fifth Street, Suite 203
  Tucson, Arizona 85716

ARKANSAS

American Diabetes Association
Arkansas Affiliate, Inc.
  5422 West Markham
  Little Rock, Arkansas 72205

CALIFORNIA

American Diabetes Association
Northern California Affiliate, Inc.

255 Hugo Street
San Francisco, California 94122
American Diabetes Association
Northern California Affiliate, Inc.

[Alameda–Contra Costa Chapter]
  4383 Piedmont Avenue
  Oakland, California 94611
[Marin County Chapter]
  Sierra Building
  1368 Lincoln Avenue, Room 105
  San Rafael, California 94901

[Sacramento Chapter]
  Central Methodist Church
  5265 H Street
  Sacramento, California 95819
[San Mateo Chapter]
  3080 La Selva, Room 26
  San Mateo, California 94403
American Diabetes Association
Southern California Affiliate, Inc.
  1127 Crenshaw Boulevard
  Los Angeles, California 90019

[San Diego Chapter]
  3420 Kenyon Street, Suite 240
  San Diego, California 92110
[Orange County Chapter]
  1215 East Chapman Avenue, Suite 4D
  Orange, California 92666

COLORADO

American Diabetes Association
Colorado Affiliate, Inc.
  1045 Acoma Street
  Denver, Colorado 80204

CONNECTICUT

American Diabetes Association
Connecticut Affiliate, Inc.
  17 Oakwood Avenue
  West Hartford, Connecticut 06119

DELAWARE

American Diabetes Association
Delaware Affiliate, Inc.
  2300 Pennsylvania Avenue, Suite LL1
  Wilmington, Delaware 19806

DISTRICT OF COLUMBIA

American Diabetes Association
Washington, D.C. Area Affiliate, Inc.
  7961 Eastern Avenue
  Silver Spring, Maryland 20910

FLORIDA

American Diabetes Association
Florida Affiliate, Inc.
  1080 Woodcock Road, Suite 279
  Orlando, Florida 32803

GEORGIA

American Diabetes Association
Georgia Affiliate, Inc.
  1447 Peachtree Street, N.E., Suite 810
  Atlanta, Georgia 30309

HAWAII

American Diabetes Association
Hawaii Affiliate, Inc.
  347 North Kuakini Street
  Honolulu, Hawaii 96817

IDAHO

American Diabetes Association
Idaho Affiliate, Inc.
  P.O. Box 7113
  Boise, Idaho 83707

ILLINOIS

American Diabetes Association
Northern Illinois Affiliate, Inc.
  620 North Michigan Avenue
  Chicago, Illinois 60611
American Diabetes Association
Downstate Illinois Affiliate, Inc.
  104 North Water, Room 623
  Decatur, Illinois 62523

INDIANA

American Diabetes Association
Indiana Affiliate, Inc.
  222 S. Downey Avenue, Suite 320
  Indianapolis, Indiana 46219
[Greater Indianapolis Chapter]
  1433 North Meridian Street
  Indianapolis, Indiana 46202

IOWA

American Diabetes Association
Iowa Affiliate, Inc.
  305 Second Avenue, S.E.
  Cedar Rapids, Iowa 52401

KANSAS

American Diabetes Association
Kansas Affiliate, Inc.
  2312 East Central
  Wichita, Kansas 67214

KENTUCKY

American Diabetes Association
Kentucky Affiliate, Inc.
  2358 Pierson Drive
  Lexington, Kentucky 40505

LOUISIANA

American Diabetes Association
Louisiana Affiliate, Inc.
   619 Jefferson Highway, Suite 1F
   Baton Rouge, Louisiana 70816

MAINE

See Massachusetts.

MARYLAND

American Diabetes Association
Maryland Affiliate, Inc.
   3701 Old Court Road
   Old Court Executive Park, Suite 19
   Baltimore, Maryland 21208

MASSACHUSETTS

American Diabetes Association
New England Affiliate, Inc.
   377 Elliot Street
   Newton Upper Falls, Massachusetts
   02164

MICHIGAN

American Diabetes Association
Michigan Affiliate, Inc.
   6131 West Outer Drive
   Detroit, Michigan 48235

MINNESOTA

American Diabetes Association
Minnesota Affiliate, Inc.
   5400 Glenwood Avenue North
   Minneapolis, Minnesota 55422
[Twin Cities Chapter]
   5400 Glenwood Avenue North
   Minneapolis, Minnesota 55422

MISSISSIPPI

American Diabetes Association
Mississippi Affiliate, Inc.
   P.O. Box 16968
   Jackson, Mississippi 39206

MISSOURI

American Diabetes Association
Heart of America Affiliate, Inc.
   616 East 63rd Street, Suite 203
   Kansas City, Missouri 64110
American Diabetes Association
Missouri Regional Affiliate, Inc.
   Box 11
   Columbia, Missouri 65201
American Diabetes Association
Greater St. Louis Affiliate, Inc.
   3839 Lindell Boulevard
   St. Louis, Missouri 63108

MONTANA

American Diabetes Association
Montana Affiliate, Inc.
   Box 2411
   Great Falls, Montana 59403

NEBRASKA

American Diabetes Association
Nebraska Affiliate, Inc.
   819 Dorcas Street
   Omaha, Nebraska 68108

NEVADA

American Diabetes Association
Nevada Affiliate, Inc.
   3333 West Washington Avenue
   Las Vegas, Nevada 89107

NEW HAMPSHIRE

American Diabetes Association
New Hampshire Affiliate, Inc.
   P.O. Box 1312
   Concord, New Hampshire 03301

NEW JERSEY

American Diabetes Association
New Jersey Affiliate, Inc.
   American Red Cross Building
   345 Union Street
   Hackensack, New Jersey 07601

NEW MEXICO

American Diabetes Association
New Mexico Affiliate, Inc.
  6101 Marble, N.E., Suite 11
  Albuquerque, New Mexico 87110

NEW YORK

American Diabetes Association
Upper Hudson Area Chapter, Inc.
  35 Hackett Avenue
  Albany, New York 12205
American Diabetes Association
Western New York Affiliate, Inc.
  Statler Hilton
  107 Delaware Avenue, Suite 240
  Buffalo, New York 14202
American Diabetes Association
New York Diabetes Affiliate, Inc.
  104 East 40th Street
  New York, New York 10016
Rochester Regional Diabetes Association,
Inc.
  1351 Mount Hope Avenue, Room 121
  Rochester, New York 14620
American Diabetes Association
Upstate New York Chapter, Inc.
  710 Wilson Building
  306 South Salina Street
  Syracuse, New York 13202
American Diabetes Association
Central New York Chapter, Inc.
  1404 Genesee Street
  Utica, New York 13502

NORTH CAROLINA

American Diabetes Association
North Carolina Affiliate, Inc.
  408 North Tryon Street
  Charlotte, North Carolina 28202

NORTH DAKOTA

American Diabetes Association
North Dakota Affiliate, Inc.
  P.O. Box 234
  Grand Forks, North Dakota 58201

OHIO

American Diabetes Association
Akron Area Affiliate, Inc.
  225 West Exchange Street
  Akron, Ohio 44302
American Diabetes Association
Cincinnati Affiliate, Inc.
  2400 Reading Road
  Cincinnati, Ohio 45202
American Diabetes Association
Dayton Area Affiliate, Inc.
  184 Salem Avenue
  Dayton, Ohio 45406
American Diabetes Association
Mahoning Valley Chapter, Inc.
  420 Oak Hill Avenue
  Youngstown, Ohio 44502
American Diabetes Association
Southeastern Ohio Chapter, Inc.
  Box 2354
  Zanesville, Ohio 43701

OKLAHOMA

American Diabetes Association
Eastern Oklahoma Chapter, Inc.
  6565 South Yale Avenue, Suite 613
  Tulsa, Oklahoma 74136
American Diabetes Association
Western Oklahoma Chapter, Inc.
  2801 N.W. Expressway, Suite 146
  Oklahoma City, Oklahoma 73112

OREGON

American Diabetes Association
Oregon Affiliate, Inc.
  3607 S.W. Corbett
  Portland, Oregon 97201

PENNSYLVANIA

American Diabetes Association
Greater Philadelphia Affiliate, Inc.
  919 Walnut Street, Fourth Floor
  Philadelphia, Pennsylvania 19107
American Diabetes Association
Western Pennsylvania Affiliate, Inc.
  4401 5th Avenue
  Pittsburgh, Pennsylvania 15213

American Diabetes Association
Pennsylvania Affiliate, Inc.
739 Hamilton Mall, Room 303
Allentown, Pennsylvania 18101

RHODE ISLAND

See Massachusetts.

SOUTH CAROLINA

American Diabetes Association
South Carolina Affiliate, Inc.
P.O. Box 6562
745 No. Pleasantburg Drive
Greenville, South Carolina 29606

SOUTH DAKOTA

American Diabetes Association
South Dakota Affiliate, Inc.
P.O. Box 1842
Aberdeen, South Dakota 57401

TENNESSEE

American Diabetes Association
Greater Chattanooga Chapter, Inc.
871 McCallie Avenue
Chattanooga, Tennessee 37403
American Diabetes Association
Knox Area Unit, Inc.
815 Broadway, N.E.
Knoxville, Tennessee 37917
American Diabetes Association
Memphis Mid-South Chapter, Inc.
969 Madison Avenue, Suite 900-A
Memphis, Tennessee 38104
American Diabetes Association
Middle Tennessee Chapter, Inc.
c/o Baptist Hospital
Room 120, West Building
2000 Church Street
Nashville, Tennessee 37236

TEXAS

American Diabetes Association
North Texas Affiliate, Inc.
P.O. Box 35785 (Mailing Address)

5415 Maple, Suite 216
Dallas, Texas 75235
American Diabetes Association
South Texas Affiliate, Inc.
1536 East Anderson Lane, Suite 36
Austin, Texas 78711
[Capital Area Chapter]
4101 Medical Parkway #104
Austin, Texas 78765
[Greater Houston Area Chapter]
2990 Richmond, Suite 100
Houston, Texas 77098

UTAH

American Diabetes Association
Utah Affiliate, Inc.
Graystone Plaza, #4
1174 East 2700 South
Salt Lake City, Utah 84106

VERMONT

American Diabetes Association
Vermont Affiliate, Inc.
106 Colchester Avenue
Burlington, Vermont 05401

VIRGINIA

American Diabetes Association
Virginia Affiliate, Inc.
Suite 5, 210 Laskin Road
Virginia Beach, Virginia 23451

WASHINGTON

American Diabetes Association
Washington Affiliate, Inc.
1218 Terry Avenue, Suite 209
Seattle, Washington 98101
[Anchorage Unit]
8130 Huckleberry
Anchorage, Alaska 99502

WEST VIRGINIA

American Diabetes Association
West Virginia Affiliate, Inc.
1036 Quarrier Street, Room 404
Charleston, West Virginia 25301

WISCONSIN	WYOMING
American Diabetes Association	American Diabetes Association
Wisconsin Affiliate, Inc.	Wyoming Affiliate, Inc.
P.O. Box 17805 (Mailing Address)	DePaul Hospital
5215 North Ironwood Road	2600 East 18th
Milwaukee, Wisconsin 53217	Cheyenne, Wyoming 82001

Index

185

About the Author

Angela Bowen is a graduate of Mississippi State University and the University of Washington School of Medicine. She completed a Fellowship in Metabolic Diseases at Virginia Mason Medical Center in Seattle and has been active in diabetes research since 1964. She is a past president of the Washington Diabetes Association and has served on the Food and Nutrition Committee of the American Diabetes Association. She is also a past president of her local medical society and is currently serving as president of the Washington Society of Internal Medicine. Her current research is supported by the Olympia-Tumwater Foundation. She has a private practice in Olympia, Washington, where she lives with her husband, Jack Brennan.